English-Chinese Laboratory Manual for Medical Physiology

英汉对照·医学生理学实验指导

主编　彭碧文　张先荣

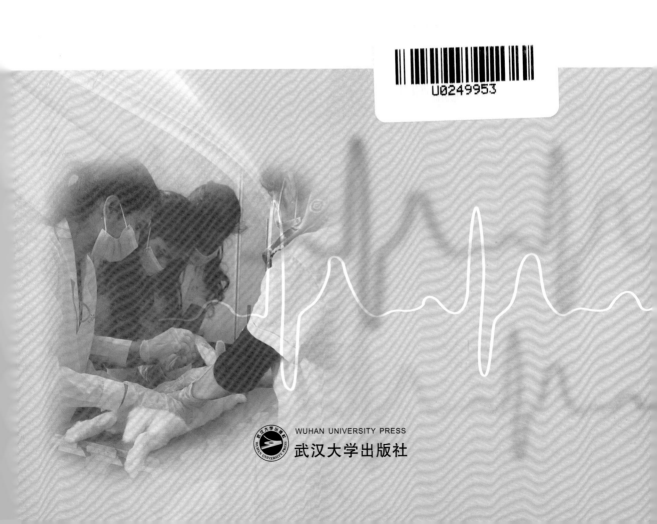

WUHAN UNIVERSITY PRESS
武汉大学出版社

图书在版编目(CIP)数据

医学生理学实验指导:英汉对照/彭碧文,张先荣主编. —武汉:武汉大学出版社,2018.10

ISBN 978-7-307-20183-5

Ⅰ.医… Ⅱ.①彭… ②张… Ⅲ.人体生理学—医学院校—教学参考资料—英、汉 Ⅳ.R33

中国版本图书馆 CIP 数据核字(2018)第 098207 号

责任编辑:谢文涛　　　责任校对:汪欣怡　　　版式设计:韩闻锦

出版发行:**武汉大学出版社**　(430072　武昌　珞珈山)

(电子邮件:cbs22@whu.edu.cn　网址:www.wdp.com.cn)

印刷:湖北金海印务有限公司

开本:787×1092　1/16　印张:12.5　字数:289 千字　插页:1

版次:2018 年 10 月第 1 版　　2018 年 10 月第 1 次印刷

ISBN 978-7-307-20183-5　　定价:36.00 元

Contents

目　　录

Preface

1. An Overview of Physiology Experiments

Physiological experiments observe the changes of the function and metabolism of the organisms, mainly on animals and the human body, under the conditions of normal or with chemical compound treatments, thus to explore mechanism and regularity.

The main target of physiological experiments is to explain the physical and chemical factors that are responsible for the origin, development, and progression of life based on *in vitro* or *in vivo* experiments. It is beneficial for students to understand the process of life activities, diseases, and treatment. Physiological experiments have become a basic compulsory course in medical science which involves the theories and the experimental techniques of pharmacology, pathophysiology, statistics, zoology and computer science. This overview systematically introduces the basic knowledge of the physiological experiments including the basic theory, experimental methods, modern experimental techniques and experimental research. Hopefully it can cultivate the students' ability of utilizing knowledge and scientific practice through the foundation, comprehensive experiments.

2. The Rules of Laboratory

①Observe the discipline and arrive at the lab on time. Exemption from attending the course should be applied for.

②Wear lab coats in the laboratory at all time, otherwise you are not allowed to enter.

③Work seriously and earnestly while doing experiments, do not engage in any other activities that are not related to the experiments.

④Speak with a lower voice and keep quiet while you are in the laboratory. Eating and drinking are not allowed in the laboratory.

⑤ The experimental animals and equipments will be issued by groups. Any want of supplements should be allowed by teachers.

⑥The experimental instruments and equipments in each group should be used by yourselves and any replacements are not allowed in case of disorders.

⑦If an instrument is out of order, please report to the teacher in charge of the class so as to repair or replace it as soon as possible. Do not try to conceal the truth, let alone dissemble or repair it by yourself. You should compensate for the breakdown of any instrument due to violation of operating procedures.

⑧After the experiments, please wash and wipe the surgical instruments, clean up the laboratory equipment, supplies, and your experiment table. The number of equipment and supplies must be counted clearly, do not make a mess of them. Animal bodies, wastes, and scraps of paper should be put to the designated location, littering is not allowed here. After the class, the students on duty should clean the laboratory floor and check the safety of it.

⑨Writing reports on experiments would be required to submit on time. Normally your experimental reports will be submitted to the teacher in charge of the class within one week of the completion of the experiments and your sheets handed in will be concerned in final examination marks.

(Peng Biwen)

3. Methods of Writing an Experimental Report

(1) Purpose of Writing an Experimental Report

The experimental report is a summary of an experiment and also a basic training of the experimental class. By writing the experiment reports, you learn the basic format of scientific paper writing and basic methods of chart drawing, data analysis, and literature reviewing, as well as using the experimental data and literature to analyze and summarize the results of the experiment and improve the your ability to analyze, hypothesis and summarize the problems, thus laying a good foundation for future scientific paper writing.

(2) Requirements of Writing an Experimental Report

You are supposed to hold a scientific attitude when writing the experimental reports and finish them seriously and earnestly all by yourself. You shouldn't blindly copy books and experimental reports of others. Meanwhile, you ought to pay attention to making your words and sentences concise and smooth, as well as making your handwriting clear and clean, you should always keep in minds to use the punctuations correctly.

(3) General format and notice of Writing an Experimental Report

The experimental report of physiology

Name   Student number   Class   Group   Date

The title of experiment

A title can highly summarize the central idea and main content of an experimental report, which should be concise and comprehensive. You can use the title in this textbook. Remember to add the sequence number on every experimental item.

The purpose of experiment

At the beginning of an experimental report, you can raise more than one problem that the experiment should resolve. Remember that refinement and simplicity are both required.

Materials and methods of experiment

The materials and methods reported in the experiment are generally formatted as follows:

①Objects: Type, strain, gender and physical station of experimental animals. gender, body weight, and age of human body.

②Instruments: Name and manufacturer of instruments components and parameters of experimental instrument system.

③Drugs and reagents: Name, specification, dosage forms, and manufacturer of drugs and reagents.

④Experimental procedure: experimental environment and conditions, preparation methods of samples, rearing condition for experimental animals, preparation methods of drugs and reagents. Grouping and handling of experimental subjects, the experimental procedures and processes, operating methods and so on.

⑤Analysis of data: Observation methods data recording and collection of information and results.

⑥Statistical analysis

Results

Results include table, chart, and text narrative and so forth. You shall provide the following content in experimental results:

①Text description of the results

②The original experimental data in a manner of table.

③A chart or a table after statistical processing.

④Original recording curves through editing and marking

⑤The text description of your diagram and table.

Discussion and conclusion

The experimental results are discussed according to the known theoretical knowledge to explain and analyze the results. The analysis should point out the theoretical or practical significance of the experimental results. If any unexpected result occurs, you should consider and analyze the possible reasons of it and write them in your discussion.

The conclusion is a general judgment summarized from your experimental results and discussion, i. e a concise summary of concepts or theories that can be verified by this experiment. The conclusion should correspond with the purpose of this experiment. You should write your conclusion concisely. Neither should you list the specific results nor infer or extend your conclusion too far. Theoretical analysis that fails to obtain sufficient evidence in the experimental results should not be written in your conclusion.

References

You are supposed to choose the latest published books or papers closely related to methods, results and discussions in the experimental reports.

(Peng Biwen)

Chapter 1　Biological Signal Recording System

RM6240 Physiological Signal Recording System

1. 1　The Characteristics of RM6240

RM6240 Physiological signal recording systems (including RM6240B and RM6240C) are a new generation of medical and laboratory instruments produced by the Chengdu Instrument Factory. The RM6240 has two ports including an Enhanced Parallel Port (EPP) and a USB with a 12-bit A/D converter. The sampling frequency can achieve as high as 100kHz (EPP) or 200kHz (PCI high speed type).

This system is equipped with a multichannel and multifunctional amplifier. The amplifier in each channel has the function of a bioelectric amplifier, blood pressure amplifier, or bridge amplifier. It can also be used as a lung monitor (supplied with flow transducer), a thermometer (supplied with temperature transducer), and a pH meter (supplied with pH probe amplifier). In addition, this system also provides other functions, such as a drop recorder, sounder recorder, and a program-controlled and isolated stimulator.

1. 2　Instrument Panel

(1) Channel input port. The channel is a physical path for analog signal input, signal amplification, digital signal conversion, and signal recording. RM6240B can process and record sync signals from 4 channels.

(2) Stimulator output port. Output voltage or current stimulation with a square waveform.

(3) Drop recorder input. Signals of drops can be input through this channel when connected with a drop collector and detector. This input port can also be used for recording external trigger signals.

(4) Sound recorder input. Sound signals from allocated channel can be recorded when it is connected with the sound box.

1. 3   The Windows User Interface

The user interface of the RM6240 recording system can be divided into 6 functional areas:

(1) Menu. Top-level menu is located at the top of the window. Selecting either one of them will activate the drop down menu.

(2) Tool Bar. The toolbar is displayed across the top of the application window, below the menu bar. The toolbar provides quick mouse access to many tools used in the Menu.

(3) Parameter control area. Parameters for each channel are found in this area, including channel mode, scanning rate, sensitivity, and cut-off frequency. These parameters can be adjusted by selecting the corresponding button.

(4) Data display area. Data will be shown in waveform in this area.

(5) Ruler and Data Processing. This area is located on the left side of the window, its shows the number of each channel and corresponding ruler. Click the "Processing" button in this area, it will activate the drop down menu which shows channel calibration, marker, measurement and analysis, data processing, et al.

(6) Stimulator. The parameters of the program-controlled stimulator can be adjusted in the floating pop-up window.

1. 4   The Basic Function

1. 4. 1   Instrument Parameters

1. Shortcut for setting parameters

Parameters for most of the experiment program have been properly set. Start RM6240 software, select the program needed in the "experiment" menu bar, and the parameters will be set automatically according to the experiment.

2. Parameters for amplifier

(1) Selection of channel mode: click "channel mode" and select the form of recorded signal in drop down menu.

(2) Bandpass setting

Time constant: specify a system's low-frequency response.

High-frequency filter: adjust the high-frequency cutoff.

(3) Sampling rate. Sampling rate ranges from 1Hz to 100kHz. Appropriate sampling rate should be selected according to the frequency of signals in the experiment. Choose high

sampling rate when the frequency of signals are high, and low sampling rate when the frequency of signals are low.

(4) Sensitivity. Display the signals in appropriate amplitude by adjusting the sensitivity in order to record and analyze data properly.

1. 4. 2   Signal Recording

1. Shortcut for Signal Recording
There are four functional shortcut buttons for signal recording:

(1) Oscillography button. Start oscillography. Signals will be displayed in "signal recording area" on the current screen. System parameter adjustments can be done under the state of oscillography, but data cannot be saved in this state.

(2) Recording button. Start recording, signals will be displayed and saved.

(3) Pause button. After clicking on this button, signal recordings and saving will be paused and will continue after clicking on the "recording button" again.

(4) Stop button. After licking on this button, signal recordings and saving will be stopped. The recorded signals will be displayed in the "signal displaying area". If clicking on the "recording button" again, signals will be recorded and saved in another page (the signals in different pages can be displayed on the screen by pressing the "Page Up" and " Page Down" key).

2. Triggering of Synchronizing Record
Open stimulator window, select "Synchronizer trigger", click "start stimulation" button to record and display signals. Signals will be displayed on one "screen" from left to right. The number of displaying "screen" of signals is based on the "repetition" times of stimulation.

1. 4. 3   Stimulator

When stimulation is needed in a certain experiment, select stimulator, select stimulating mode, adjust stimulation parameters.

1. Function Palette
(1) Synchronizer trigger. Once choosing "synchronizer trigger", signal recording and stimulating pulse will be processed synchronously. The system will display signals in one "screen" in response to each stimulation.

(2) Record current waveform. The waveform on the current screen will be saved in a subfile. T waveform will be displayed once on "screen" in response to clicking on the button, and will be saved in a separate subfile.

(3) Non-superimposing. The newly recorded original waveform will be displayed on one "screen" in response to each stimulation.

(4) Superposed average. The waveform evoked by the current stimulation will be superposed with all waveforms recorded before by the synchronizer trigger and averaged. The averaged waveform will be displayed on the screen.

(5) Superposed accumulation. The waveform evoked by the current stimulation will be superposed with all waveforms recorded before by the synchronizer trigger, the superposed waveform will be displayed on the screen.

(6) Start stimulation. After clicking on this button, the stimulator will output stimulation pulses according to the mode and parameters set on the panel.

(7) Stop stimulation. After clicking on this button, the stimulator will stop outputting stimulation pulses.

2. Stimulation Parameters

The output stimulation pulse from the stimulator is a square wave. The basic parameters are as follow:

(1) Stimulation intensity. The intensity of voltage or current of the output pulse. The range of the output voltage is from 0 to 50 volts. The increment of it is 0.02V between 0 and 10V, and 0.05V between 10 and 50V. The range of output current is from 0 to 10 mA.

(2) Pulse width. Time interval between the leading edge and trailing edge of a square pulse. It is the duration of stimulation. It can be modulated from 0.1 to 1000ms.

(3) Pulse interval. Time interval of inter-pulse in continuous pulse stimulation. It can be modulated between 0.1 and 1000ms. The reciprocal of the sum of the pulse width and pulse interval is stimulation frequency, ranging from 1 to 3000Hz.

(4) Major cycle. The stimulator outputs sequential pulses per unit time. Stimulation pulses can be one, a few, or even several hundred in a single major cycle, and pulse interval varies and can be set as needed. "Number of cycle" or "repetitive times" refers to the numbers of periodic output stimulation per "major cycle". For example, when "major cycle" = 1s, "number of pulse" = 3, "delay" = 5ms, "pulse interval" = 200ms, "pulse width" = 1ms, "stimulation intensity" = 1v, "repetitive times" = 7. Click the "stimulation button" and the stimulator will output stimulations at 1V intensity, 3 pulses with 1ms "pulse width", "pulse width" 200ms. The first pulse will begin at 5ms of stimulation, and the stimulation will be repeated for 7 times. The major cycle, delay, pulse width, pulse interval, and number of pulses should be set in line with the following formula: major cycle (s) > delay (s) + [pulse width (s) + pulse interval (s)] × number of pulse.

(5) Number of pulse. The number of pulses output from the stimulator in a set period.

(6) Delay. The period from the time when the stimulator starts to the time when the pulse output. The delay can be used to adjust the level of signals on screen when using triggering of synchronizing recording.

3. Output Mode

Stimulator can output constant voltage or constant current. It delivers a pulse that is rectangular in shape. The constant voltage may have positive or negative voltage output pulse. The constant current also has positive or negative current output pulse.

4. Stimulation Mode

A pulse sequence can be made up with a series of parameters, such as a certain major cycle, number of pulses, pulse interval, etc. This specific pulse sequence is called stimulation mode. The basic stimulation modes are as following, meeting the needs of most experiments.

(1) Single twitch stimulation. Only one stimulation pulse is output in a major cycle. The adjustable parameters are intensity, pulse width, delay, major cycle, and repetitive times. The signals can be caught in the triggering of synchronizing recording. This stimulation mode is used mostly in recording compound action potential in a nerve trunk, a single twitch of skeletal muscle, premature contraction, evoked potential, etc.

(2) Continuous single stimulation. The major cycle is 1s, and the stimulation is recycled unlimitedly. The number of pulses output in a major cycle is frequency, and the pulse intervals are equal. The stimulation mode is always used when stimulating the depressor nerve and vagus nerve, as well as recording the effect of the stimulating frequency on skeletal muscle contraction.

(3) Double stimulation. Two stimulation pulses are output in a major cycle. The adjustable parameters are intensity, pulse width, delay, pulse interval, major cycle, and repetitive numbers. The signals can be caught in triggering of synchronizing recording. This mode can be used in recording skeletal muscle contraction, or in a refractory period recording experiment.

(4) Train stimulation. A series of stimulation will be output in a major cycle, the number of pulses ranging from 3 to 999. The adjustable parameters are intensity, pulse width, delay, pulse interval, major cycle, number of pulses, repetitive times. The triggering of synchronizing recording is applicable in this stimulation mode. This mode can be used in stimulating the depressor nerve or vagus nerve, as well as recording the effect of stimulation frequency on skeletal muscle contraction.

(5) Timed stimulation. The stimulating pulse will be output according to the set frequency in a given stimulation time. It is usually used when observing the effect of stimulation frequency in the same stimulation time. For example, stimulating the depressor nerve or vagus nerve, as well as the effect of stimulation frequency on skeletal muscle contraction. The adjustable parameters are delay, pulse width, amplitude, time, frequency, major cycle, and repetitive times.

(6) Stimulation intensity increases or decreases automatically. Under single twitch or double stimulation mode, the stimulation intensity automatically increases or decreases with a certain increment from initial intensity. This mode is used for automatic testing of stimulation intensity and response.

(7) Stimulation frequency ascending or descending automatically. Under single twitch or timed stimulation mode, the stimulation frequency automatically increases or decreases with a

certain increment from initial frequency. This mode is used for automatic testing of stimulation intensity and response.

(8) Pulse width increases or decreases automatically. Under single twitch or continuous single stimulation mode, the stimulation pulse width automatically increases or decreases with a certain increment from initial pulse width. This mode is used for automatic testing of basic intensity and timing.

(9) Double train stimulation. Two stimulation pulses form a group of pulses in this mode; a few to several hundred of pulse groups can be output in one major cycle. The adjustable parameters are intensity, pulse width, delay, pulse interval, frequency, group numbers, major cycle, and repetitive times.

(10) Continuous double stimulation. Continuous double stimulation is essentially the same as double train stimulation. The groups of pulses in a major cycle can be expressed in frequency.

(11) Advanced function. Stimulation train can be further specialized by modulating parameters, such as major cycle, intensity, pulse interval, the number of pulse, et al. It is called 'programmed stimulator'.

(Zhang Xianrong)

Chapter 2   Basic Laboratory Techniques
of Physiology

2. 1   Basic Knowledge of Laboratory Animals

2. 1. 1   Classification for Laboratory Animals

Clear biological characteristics and genetic background are required for laboratory animals. Furthermore, pathogens and parasites in animals should be strictly controlled.

1. Genetic classification of Laboratory Animals

(1) Inbred strains of animals. For these animals, the usual procedure is mating of brother-sister pairs for 20 generations. Animals of an inbred strain can be expected to be homozygous at 98. 6 percent of their loci. The continuous overlaying of similar genetics exposes recessive gene patterns that often lead to changes in reproduction performance and ability to survive.

(2) Outbred strains of animals. These animals are closed colonies of animals that are not uniformly homozygous, that is, they are not inbred. The primary objective in the maintenance of an outbred strain is to ensure that the strain remains constant in all characteristics for as many generations as possible.

(3) F1 hybrids. An F1 hybrid is a first generation cross between two inbred strains. Individual F1 hybrids of a specific cross are genetically identical to one another, but are heterozygous at all alleles in which the parental strains differed. F1 hybrids are more vigorous than inbred strains. F1 hybrids are highly homogenous, as their phenotypes are extremely uniform and predictable.

2. Classification According to Pathogen Control

(1) Conventional animals. Conventional animals are housed under natural conditions, whose microbial burden is unknown and uncontrolled; however, these animals are free of amphixenosis pathogens. Parasites and germs are permitted in these animals.

(2) Clean-class animals. Clean-class animals are housed in a low-security barrier and demonstrated to be free of major pathogens, such as amphixenosis pathogens and external parasites.

(3) Specific pathogen free animals. SPF animals are designated to be free from specified pathogens. SPF animals are only free from tested specific pathogens, however the hidden/unknown pathogens are usually overlooked.

(4) Germfree animals. Germfree rodents are free of all aerobic and anaerobic organisms with the possible exception of endogenous viruses. Germfree, or axenic, animals are generally maintained in semi-rigid isolators. All supplies are sterilized and entered into the isolator using strict gnotobiotic techniques.

2.1.2   Species and Characteristics of Animals

(1) Toad and frog. The toad and frog are amphibians belonging to the order Anura. Some of their basic life activities are similar to that of homothermal animals. In addition, the in vitro culture condition for their tissue or organ is simple and easily controlled. Therefore, toad and frog are widely used in research and teaching in physiology.

(2) Rabbit. Rabbits are small mammals of the order Rodentia, they are also classified in the order Lagomorpha. The housed rabbits are generally docile and easy to handle for oral gavage or blood collecting. A marginal ear vein is always used for intravenous injection due to its superficial location. The sinus and aortic depressor nerve in the rabbit is separated from the vagus nerve and sympathetic nerve, therefore, it is used for several experiments such as regulation of cardiovascular activity, regulation of respiration, and renal regulation of urine volume. In addition, the rabbit's digestive activities are active and have typical physiological characteristics; the digestive tract is used for studying general characteristics of smooth muscle and its function.

(3) Mouse and Rat. The mouse and rat are both mammals of the Rodentia order. Laboratory rats or mice have been widely used in scientific research, have served as an important animal model for research in medicine, pharmacology, oncology, genetics, immunology, and other various types of disease. The physiological locations in the rat brain areas are clear and have been normalized; the rat brain is widely used in neuroscience research.

(4) Guinea pig. The guinea pig, also called the "cavy", is a species of rodent belonging to the family Caviidae. It's hearing has been highly developed and it is very keen. In addition, the structure of the guinea pig ear is similar to that of humans. Guinea pigs are therefore a preferred animal model for studying the auditory system.

2.1.3   Laboratory Animal Selection

Laboratory animal selection has important implications for the quality of research. To choose laboratory animals, the following rules should be considered.

（1）Similarity principles. Choose those animals which have similar characteristics of physiological function, metabolism and signs of the disease to meet the experiments' needs.

（2）Standardizing principles. Choose appropriate species, strain and microbiological background of the animal, as well as standard breeding conditions. The animals' age, weight, gender, and health condition should be consistent.

（3）Economization principles. Use the most cost effective and easily-housed animals.

2. 1. 4 Handling and Restraint of Animals

Animals should be fixed on the dissection board properly after anesthesia, which allows the animals to undergo surgery and other procedures without the distress. Generally, the animals are fixed on the dissection board in supine position. This position applies to the surgery in the neck, thorax, abdomen, and thigh. Prone position applies to the surgery in the brain and spinal cord.

（1）Rabbit. Grasp the loose skin around the neck with one hand and using your other hand or arm, support the rabbit's hind quarters. The rabbit's hind end should be supported immediately after removal from its cage. If the rabbit is held properly, it will feel secure and will not struggle.

（2）Mouse and Rat. Grab the rat by the base of the tail and lift out of the cage and place over the wire bar lid of the cage. Use your right hand to pull the tail backward, while the mouse or rat will try to crawl forward. Grasp the loose skin behind its neck with your left thumb and forefinger, hold the tail and support the lower body with your right hand, or secure the tail with the same hand（left ring and little fingers）. Care should be taken that if the rat will react violently to restraint, thick gloves or clothes will be useful to avoid getting bitten.

（3）Guinea pig. Guinea pigs are not aggressive by nature. Calmly grasp it with one hand under the chest and use your other hand to support its hindquarters.

（4）Toad and frog. Use your thumb, index finger and middle finger to control the fore legs, and use your ring finger and little finger to control the hind legs.

2. 2 Methods for Reagents Administration

2. 2. 1 Oral Administration

（1）Administration by mouse. Put the stable water-soluble reagents into the drinking water of the animals, or mix the water insoluble reagents into animal food. Animals will take the reagents spontaneously. The animal will be in a natural state during oral administration. This method will not induce stress in the animal and apply to chronic pharmacological treatment in animal experiments. The disadvantage of this method is that it is difficult to ensure the correct dosage because of inter individual difference in drinking and food intake amount, which will influence the accuracy of the effect reagents.

(2) Administration by oral gavage. Liquid compounds can be administrated directly into the stomach of mice or rat via oral gavage. Restrain the animal and maintain the animal in an upright position with the left hand. With the right hand hold the gavage needle, passing the gavage needle along the side of the mouse. Advance the needle into the esophagus and toward the stomach. After the needle is passed to the correct length, the compound may be slowly injected. If the animal coughs, chokes, or begins to struggle after the compound administration begins you may be injecting material into the lungs. If resistance is encountered you may be attempting to enter the trachea and you should withdraw the needle and alter your needle position.

2.2.2   Administration by Injection

(1) Subcutaneous injection. The reagent is administered into the layer of skin directly below the dermis and epidermis; it applies to all mammals. Restrain the animal, lift the skin with your fingers to make a "tent", and insert the needle into the subcutaneous tissue. You may move the tip of needle around slightly. The needle is in a subcutaneous area if it is easy to move. Aspirate prior to injection to make sure the needle is not in a vessel.

(2) Intramuscular injection. Intramuscular injection applies to almost all water-soluble and insoluble reagents. The reagent is injected directly into a muscle, which has plentiful blood supply. Reagents can be absorbed quickly and reach the systemic circulation. In the rat and other small rodents, the very small muscle mass makes intramuscular injection technically difficult. If intramuscular injections are necessary, they can be made into the back of the thigh in all small rodents. Restrain the animal in an appropriate way and direct the needle through the skin into muscle belly. Aspiration should be attempted before injection to determine the accidental penetration of a blood vessel has not occurred.

(3) Intraperitoneal injection. Intraperitoneal injection is the most frequently performed route administration in mice and rats. The large surface area of the abdominal cavity and its abundant blood supply facilitate rapid absorption. Intraperitoneal injections should be administered in the lower right or left quadrant of the abdomen to avoid vital organs. Rat or mice should be restrained and held with the ventrum exposed and head pointed downward, allowing the freely moveable abdominal organs to fall out of the way. The needle should be directed towards the animal's head at an angle of 20-30° degrees. To avoid intestine or urinary bladder injection, it is essential to insert only the tip of the needle into the peritoneal cavity. Aspiration should be attempted to ensure that hollow organs such as the bladder or colon, or

blood vessels have not been penetrated.

(4) Intravenous injection. Intravenous injections offer various advantages over the other routes of administration. For example, it allows for control over the rate of delivery into circulation, rapid response, etc. It is a common way of applying reagents in acute and chronic experiments. Choose an appropriate vein for injection according to structural characteristics of the animal's anatomy.

① Intravenous injection through marginal ear vein. Restrain the rabbit on the bench, remove the hair around marginal ear vein, gently tapping the ear to make the vein more visible, and disinfect the injection site with 70% ethanol. Stabilize the base of the ear between the left forefinger and middle finger, grasping the tip of the ear between the left thumb and ring finger. Hold the syringe with the right hand and insert the needle with the bevel up at a slight angle (the needle should be pushed into the vein at least 2-3 mm). Inject slowly and watch for clearing of the lumen. Incorrect positioning will result in a slight bulge in the ear or hard resistance upon injection. If this occurs, remove the needle and repeat the process proximal to the previous site. Attempt the injection starting at a slightly distal part of the vein for extra injections.

② Intravenous injection through tail vein. There are 3 main veins in a mouse (or rat) tail: one runs on the dorsal side of the tail, while the two others run laterally along each side of the tail. The lateral tail vein is more suitable for injection. Place the animal in a restraint device or an inverted beaker. Prior to injection, warm up the tail with 40-50°C water or scrub the tail with ethanol to dilate the veins. Stabilize the tail between the forefinger and thumb below the site where the needle will be inserted. Insert the needle with the bevel pointing upward at an angle of approximately 20 degrees into the vein towards the direction of the head. Incorrect positioning will result in a blanched area above the needle on the tail or hard resistance upon injection. If this occurs, remove the needle and re-insert above the first site. Attempt the injection starting at a slightly distal part of the vein for extra injections. It is quite difficult to pierce and enter the vessels in older rats whose tail skin is very tough and covered by scales.

2. 3   Methods of Anesthesia

The proper use of anesthesia in acute or chronic experiments is ethical and scientifically imperative. It blocks the perception of pain and other sensations, and allows the animals to undergo surgery and other procedures without the distress. The properties of anesthetic drugs, animal tolerance in anesthesia, and the purpose of the experiment are all factors that will affect the anesthesia and experiment. It follows that selection of the appropriate drug, dosage, and the route of administration must be evaluated in order to ensure the best anesthesia possible.

2.3.1   General Anesthesia

(1) Inhalant anesthesia. The commonly used inhalation anesthetic agent in animal anesthesia is ether. It does not have much effect on respiration and blood pressure. It is a fast-acting and short effect reagent. Ether can also be used for initial induction in aggressive animals. For anesthesia in small animals, put cotton balls soaked with ether into an inverted beaker or an airtight container, then put the animal in the container. Take the animal out of the container for further procedure right after it loses consciousness. Ether is a colorless volatile highly inflammable liquid with a distinct irritant smell. In particular, ether must be stored away from flame.

(2) Injectable anesthesia. Agents such as urethane, pentobarbital sodium salt, and chloralose are commonly available for use in animal anesthesia by intravenous or intraperitoneal injection.

2.3.2   Local Anesthesia

Local anesthetics cause reversible local anesthesia by blocking conduction in the nerves. There are two main types of local anesthesia as follows.

(1) Topical anesthesia. Topical anesthetics are available in ointments, sprays, or lotions and they can be applied to numb the surface of the skin or mucous membrane by blocking the nerves under the skin or mucous membrane. Anesthetics include tetracaine and lidocaine.

(2) Infiltration anesthesia. Infiltration anesthesia is an anesthesia induced by injecting the anesthetics directly into or around the tissues to block nerve conduction. These types of anesthetics have a local analgesic effect, but do not penetrate more deep than ordinary topical anesthetics. Anesthetics include procaine, cocaine, and lidocaine.

2.3.3   Monitoring Anesthesia

All anesthetized animals must be attended and monitored continually to assess adequate level of anesthesia. Animals that are too light will experience pain and may move during surgical procedure, and respiration and heart rate will change. If animals are too deep, all the responses or reflexes will decrease or even lose, and the cardiovascular center and respiratory center will be inhibited. There are as many acceptable methods to monitor anesthesia as there are species of animals. Certain methods are fairly common between species. These include:

(1) Respiratory rate. Good indicator of depth of anesthesia. Rapid, shallow respirations usually indicate the animal is too "light". Normal respiration rate varies among animals, consult veterinary text for normal values.

(2) Corneal reflex. Touching the edge of the cornea with a thread or a tuft of cotton results in a blink. Movement of the eyelids are an indication that the depth of anesthesia is not sufficient to undergo surgery. Once the animal has lost its corneal reflex, it is too deep.

(3) Muscle tone. Muscle tone is tested by pulling on the lower limb. Rigid tone indicates inadequate depth of anesthesia. Loss of muscle tone means that the animal becomes deeper.

(4) Toe pinch or skin pinch. Pinching the toe or foot without breaking the skin or causing any deep tissue damage will cause a pain response. Any observed movement (withdrawing the paw) indicates that the animal is not sufficiently anesthetized to do surgery. If it doesn't, it is not sensing pain.

The depth of anesthesia must be monitored carefully. The above 4 items should be monitored and considered together when judging the depth of anesthesia. An optimal anesthesia has the following signs: suppression of muscle tone and relaxation, slow and stable respiration, suppression of physiological response to stimuli, and weak or total loss of cornea reflex.

2.3.4 Points for Attention

(1) Choose the appropriate anesthetic drug, dosage, and administration route before anesthesia. Prepare moderate concentration of drug to keep proper volume for injection.

(2) When applying intravenous injection, the first 1/3 volume may be injected fast to make the animal calm down. The remaining 2/3 volume should be injected slowly while monitoring the depth of anesthesia.

(3) Once animals become too light and experience struggle or fast respiration, extra drug should be supplemented. Typically, 1/5 of the original dose is given for repeat doses.

(4) Monitor animal's body temperature and prevent heat loss. Monitor respiration and maintain a smooth airway throughout the procedure and recovery.

(5) Monitoring of normal physiologic functions must continue after surgery until the animal is completely recovered from anesthesia, and is able to hold itself in a normal upright position.

2.4 Surgical Instruments

Surgical instruments used in animal surgery are similar to that used in human surgery. There are also some instruments exclusively designed for performing animal surgery. The following summary describes some instruments which are most often used in physiology experiment.

(1) Surgical scalpel. It is used for cutting the skin or organs. There are 3 main types of scalpel blade, including rounded tip blade with a sharp blade and curved blade. Choose the

appropriate scalpel blade according to surgery site and purpose. The common method of holding a scalpel is like holding a pencil. Hold the scalpel near the blade between the thumb and the middle finger. The index finger may be placed on the top side of the instrument to control depth and force applied to the blade.

(2) Surgical scissors and rough scissors. There are 2 types of scissors: curved surgical scissors and straight surgical scissors. In physiological experiments, the straight scissors are used to make straight cuts for soft tissue, such as skin and muscle. We use curved scissors for cutting animal fur. Eye scissors are very fine, and should only be used for cutting small soft tissues, such as vessels and nerves. Scissors are most commonly held with the ring finger in one loop and the thumb in the other, using the middle finger and index finger to support the shaft. Rough scissors are ordinary scissors, which are used for cutting hard tissue, such as spinal cord, bone, or skin in toad experiments.

(3) Tissue forceps. Forceps used in surgery can be broadly divided into two types: toothed forceps and smooth forceps. It may be used for holding or lifting tissue for further dissection, cutting or suture. In general, the tooth forceps are used for lifting up some tough tissue, such as skin, subcutaneous tissue, fascia, tendon, etc. The teeth in toothed forceps aid traction and thus the tissue can be held tightly, but can also crush and perforate fragile organs or tissues. Therefore, the toothed forceps cannot be used for holding fragile organs. Smooth forceps are used for holding nerves, vessels, intestinal wall, or other fragile tissues. The handles of forceps are designed to be held like pencils to provide ease for manipulation and stability.

(4) Hemostat. It is commonly used in surgical procedures to control bleeding. It can also be used in dissecting tissue, holding, or pulling a suturing needle. The way of holding a hemostat is the same as that of holding scissors. There are a series of interlocking teeth on each handle, with the ratcheted handles able to be locked in multiple positions in order to maintain variable levels of constant pressure.

(5) Bone rongeur. Bone rongeur is used for gouging out bone, often in the skull or spinal cord.

(6) Bone drill. Bone drill is used to create holes in craniotomy.

(7) Trachea cannula. Trachea cannula is used for tracheal intubation to keep airway unobstructed in acute animal experiment.

(8) Vessel cannula. There are arterial cannulas and venous cannulas. For arterial cannulas, one end of the arterial cannula is inserted into the artery, while the other end will be connected with a blood pressure transducer, used for recording blood pressure in acute experiments. For the venous cannula, it will be fixed after inserting into the vein for administration of reagents during experiment processing.

(9) Pith needle. Pith needle is used for destroying the toad's brain and spinal cord.

(10) Glass rod. Glass rod is used for dissecting nerves or vessels.

(11) Toad's heart clip. Clamp the apex of the toad's heart when the heart is relaxed with the tip of the heart clip, with the tail of heart clip connected with the transducer.

(12) Artery clamp. Artery clamp is used for blocking blood flow.

(13) Dissecting board. It is a 20 cm × 15 cm wood board for fixing the toad or frog.

(Zhang Xianrong)

2. 5   Laboratory Operations and Techniques for Animal Experiment

2. 5. 1   Fixing the Experimental Animal

Animals should be fixed on the operating table after anesthesia. Fixing methods depend on the specific experimental context. The most frequently used fixing position is the supine position, which is suitable for operation and experiments on the neck, chest, abdomen, and thigh. The fixing method involves putting the animal on its back, using threads to tie the four animal limbs at wrist or ankle joints to the sides of operating table, and using a thread to hook two upper incisors and tie to the iron column on the front end of operating table. Another fixing position is the prone position, which is suitable for operation and experiments on the brain and spinal cord. The fixing method involves putting the animal on its abdomen, using threads to tie the four animal limbs at wrist or ankle joints to the sides of operating table whilefixing the head in a stereotaxic instrument or horseshoe-shaped head holder, or using a thread to hook upper incisors and tie to the iron column on the front end of the operating table. Lateral position is suitable for experiments involving the cochlea and kidney. This method is putting the animal conveniently on the operating table.

2. 5. 2   Cutting the Skin and Subcutaneous Tissue

The location and size of the operation incision is determined according to the objective and requirements of experiments. In order to expose the common carotid artery and cervical vagus nerve, the incision should be at the cervical midline. In order to expose the diaphragm, the incision should be at sub-xiphoid. To expose the heart, the incision should be in the midline of the chest or the left chest. To expose the bladder and ureter, the incision should be above the phalanges. Incision should be parallel to the blood vessels and organs. Make a mark when necessary. Fix and extend the skin with the thumb and forefinger. Hold a scalpel using another hand with the blade vertical to the supposed incision. Cut the skin and subcutaneous tissue till the subcutaneous fascia once with proper strength. The tissues should be cut layer by layer and in the same direction with the tissue fibers, avoiding blood vessel and nerve injury. Clamp the skin and tissues on the edge of the incision with several hemostatic forceps, making the operation field clear.

The bleeding must be stopped in time during the operation, which can not only prevent continued loss of blood, also can keep the operation field clear. Bleeding caused by small vessel injury can be stopped by pressing with warm saline-moistened gauze. Bleeding caused by big vessel injury can be stopped by clamping with hemostatic forceps and ligation. In order to avoid bleeding of muscle tissues, do blunt separation when the incision is in the same direction with muscle fibers; do both ends ligation and cut in the middle when they are not in the same direction.

Cover the wound with saline-moistened gauze to prevent tissue drying.

2.5.3　Separation of Nerve and Blood Vessel

The nerves and blood vessels are delicate tissues. Be careful, patient, and gentle during the separation. Separate the nerve first and then blood vessel, thin first and then thick ones. The separating direction should be parallel to nerve and blood vessels. When separating big nerve and blood vessels, separate connective tissue around the nerve or blood vessel using hemostatic forceps (or small forceps), then make the nerve or blood vessel free from the surrounding connective tissue using hemostatic forceps, cutting the attached connective tissue from the nerve or blood vessel when necessary. When separating small nerves or blood vessels, use a glass needle to do the separation carefully. Pay attention to maintain the natural anatomic location of the operation field. DO NOT use forceps or hemostatic forceps to clamp nerve or blood vessel. After separation, put a saline-moistened thread under the nerve or blood vessel.

2.5.4　Intubation

1. Tracheal Intubation

Tracheal intubation is useful for keeping the animal breathing, collection of exhaled gas, and detection of respiratory function, etc. The methods are as follows:

(1) Cut the skin along the neck midline between the throat and sternum, do blunt dissection of the subcutaneous muscle, expose the trachea, and put a thread under it.

(2) Cut the trachea at 1-2 cm down from the thyroid cartilage and between two cartilage rings about a third of the diameter at the front wall, and another cut about 0.5 cm long toward the head. The incision is "⊥" shaped.

(3) Clean the secretions and blood in the trachea. Insert the "Y" shaped tracheal cannula into the incision toward the lung direction. Tie the trachea and cannula together and fix the cannula by tying across the branches. (Figure 2-1).

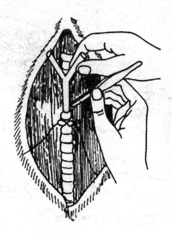

Figure 2-1   Schematic diagram of tracheal intubation

Attention:

Cervical big blood vessels and important nerves are near the neck midline. In order to avoid injury of big vessels or nerves, do blunt dissection along the muscle fiber direction when separating subcutaneous tissues.

2. Common carotid artery intubation

Common carotid artery intubation is inserting a cannula full with heparin or other anticoagulant into the common carotid artery, which is useful for blood pressure analysis and blood collection. The methods are as follows:

(1) Prepare the cannula. The insertion end is cut at an inclined plane, the other end connects with a pressure transducer. Completely fill the cannula with heparin and remove bubbles.

(2) Cut the cervical skin and subcutaneous tissues. Hold the hemostatic forceps clamping the edge of incision, lift and turn outside the cervical tissue beside trachea using the index finger of the other hand, and expose the vascular plexus.

(3) Separate the common carotid artery carefully using a glass needle and put two saline moistened threads under it.

(4) Tie the head end of the artery with a thread. Then clamp the body end of it with the artery clip. Cut the artery about 1/3-1/2 of the diameter near the ligation; the incision is 'V' shaped and at a 45 degrees angle with artery toward heart direction. Insert the cannula for about 2-3 cm into the artery toward the heart direction. Tie the artery together with the cannula and fix the cannula by tying around the branches. Remove the artery clip after you confirm that the artery is not bleeding. (Figure 2-2)

Attention:

(1) Prepare the cannula before the operation. Keep the surface smooth and full of heparin.

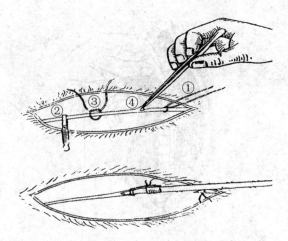

Figure 2-2   Schematic diagram of cervical artery intubation

(2) Properly cut on the artery. If too big, the artery will break; too small, it's hard to insert.

3. Common bile duct intubation

Common bile duct intubation is useful for bile secretion analysis. The methods are as follows:

(1) Cut the skin 10 cm below the xiphoid along the midline, expose the linea alba, and cut the muscle for 10 cm below the xiphoid along linea alba.

(2) Find the stomach and then duodenum, turn the duodenum down, and expose the major duodenum papilla which is connecting with the common bile duct.

(3) Put a thread under the common bile duct by using the curved needle.

(4) Cut on the major duodenum papilla. Insert the cannula for about 2-3 cm into the common bile duct toward the liver direction. Tie the duct together with a cannula and fix the cannula by tying around the branches (Figure 2-3). Yellowish-green bile will flow out immediately after insertion.

Attention:

(1) The wall of the common bile duct is thin. Prevent twisting of the cannula so as to avoid common bile duct injury or blockage of the cannula.

(2) Since there are many blood vessels in the operation area, avoiding bleeding may keep the operation field clear.

4. Ureter intubation

Ureter intubation is useful for urine formation analysis. The methods are as follows:

(1) Shear the fur above the phalanges joint, cut the skin along midline for 4-5 cm, expose the linea alba, and cut the muscle along linea alba above the phalanges joint for 5 cm.

(2) Pull the bladder outside of the abdominal cavity and turn it down. Find two ureters at

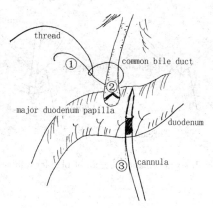

Figure 2-3   Schematic diagram of common bile duct intubation

the end of the bladder. Separate a ureter using a glass needle and put two threads under it.

(3) Tie the ureter at one end near the bladder. Cut the ureter about 1/3-1/2 of the diameter near the ligation; the incision is "V" shaped and at a 45 degrees angle with ureter toward kidney direction. Insert the cannula for about 2-3 cm into the ureter toward the kidney direction. Tie the ureter together with a cannula and fix the cannula by tying around the branches.

Attention:

(1) Prevent twisting of the cannula, so as to avoid ureter injury or blockage of the cannula.

(2) Since there are many blood vessels in the operation area, avoiding bleeding may keep the operation field clear.

5. Bladder intubation

Bladder intubation could be used for urine formation analysis. The operation is easier than ureter intubation. The methods are as follows:

(1) Pull the bladder outside of the abdominal cavity and turn it down.

(2) Urethra ligation to prevent urine flow out: put a thread below both ureters and above the urethra, turn the bladder up, and tie the urethra at the end of bladder.

(3) Clamp the top of the bladder with two hemostatic forceps, prepare a thread for fixing (Figure 2-4), make a small incision on the top of the bladder (avoid bleeding), insert the cannula for 1. 5-2 cm, tie the bladder tissue together with cannula, and fix the cannula by tying around the branches.

Attention:

(1) There are multiple layers of the bladder. DO NOT insert the cannula between the layers. The urine will flow out immediately after insertion.

(2) DO NOT insert the cannula too deep or the cannula may be blocked by tissues.

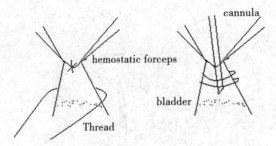

Figure 2-4   Schematic diagram of bladder intubation

2.5.5   Blood collection

The methods of blood collection are different depending on animal anatomy structure, animal size, and required blood volume.

1. Rabbit

(1) Blood collection from ear

Collect blood from marginal ear vein or central auricular artery. Shear the fur and rub the ear or swab the ear with 70% ethanol to make vasodilation. Insert a needle at an angle parallel to the artery, directed toward the base of ear. Gently aspirate with a syringe for several ml blood. Make a small incision over the vein with a needle and collect the blood as it drips from the incision. Stop bleeding by applying pressure with a cotton ball.

(2) Blood collection from femoral artery

Anesthetize and fix the rabbit with its dorsal side down on the operating table. Choose the point with most obvious arteriopalmus for puncture. Insert the needle into the artery and the blood will flow directly into the syringe. Remove the needle quickly after collection and stop bleeding.

(3) Blood collection by cardiac puncture

Anesthetize and fix the rabbit with its dorsal side down on the operating table. Shear the fur and clean the area over the xiphoid with 70% ethanol. Feel the heartbeat at the left between the third and fourth ribs. Choose the point with most obvious heartbeat for puncture. Insert needle (No. 7) into the heart and the blood will flow directly into the syringe or aspirate the syringe. Remove the needle quickly after collection and stop bleeding. The volume can reach 1/6-1/5 of total blood in rabbit. Cardiac puncture could be done again 6~7 days later.

2. Rat and mouse

(1) Blood collection from tail end

Immerse the tail in 45-50 degrees warm water to make vasodilation. Cut off tip of the tail. Squeeze from the tail root to tip. Several drops of blood could be collected.

(2) Blood collection from orbital sinus

Grasp the rat or mouse, pinching the head skin tightly using thumb and index finger to make exophthalmos. Remove an eye ball using hook small forceps. Hold the rat or mouse with head down, and the blood will flow out from the eye. The blood volume can reach 4-5% of body weight since the animal is alive, which has a heartbeat.

(3) Blood collection from posterior orbital venous plexus

Prepare the special hard glass capillary tube, length 15 cm, 1-1.5 mm in diameter, dipped in anticoagulant for a while. Grasp the rat or mouse, pinch the head skin tightly using thumb and index finger, and press both sides of the neck gently to block venous reflux. Introduce the tube end at the medial canthus of the orbit. Slowly, and with axial rotation, advance the tip of the tube gently towards the rear of the socket until blood flows into the tube. Remove the tube after collecting enough blood.

(4) Blood collection by cardiac puncture

Method is the same as in the rabbit, but the needle used can be a bit shorter.

2.5.6 Accident Treatment in Animal Experiment

Accident in animal experiment refers to the unexpected emergency, which is related to the success or failure of the experiment. Common animal experiment accidents are as follows:

1. Overdose of anesthesia

Anesthesia is a basic step in the animal operation. There are overdoses of anesthesia occasionally due to different physiological conditions of the animals. Overdose of anesthesia may cause life central paralysis, slow and irregular breathing, even breathing and heartbeat stop. In order to avoid overdose of anesthesia, operators should strictly control the speed of anesthetics injection and pay attention to the animal's breathing. Inject more slowly or stop injection when the animal breathing is too weak. Treat as soon as possible when overdose of anesthesia occurs. If the animal breathing is very slow and irregular, and a heartbeat still exists, operators should perform artificial respiration immediately. Grasp the abdomen, making it breath out, release quickly making it breath in once per second. At the same time, operators could do intravenous injection of nikethamide (50 mg/kg) which excites the respiratory center. If the animal heartbeat has stopped, operators should perform cardiac massage besides artificial respiration.

2. Hemorrhage

During the physiological experiment, hemorrhages in animals sometimes occurs due to operational errors or unforeseen reason. Prevention of experimental animal hemorrhage is very important. Operators should be familiar with the anatomical structure before the operation and be careful and patient when separating blood vessels. In cervical operation, operators should do blunt dissection of the subcutaneous muscle and connective tissue. In abdominal operation, operators should cut in the linea alba. How to treat with hemorrhage? Be calm! Find the bleeding point quickly by using cotton balls to absorb blood. Clamp both sides of the bleeding point with hemostatic forceps immediately. If the point is not too big, the bleeding will stop after a while even with hemostatic forceps removed. If the point is big, ligate both sides after the clamping. If bleeding is caused by the carotid artery cannula loosened or vessel puncture by the cannula, do intubation again after ligation or bleeding stop.

3. Asphyxia

Asphyxia refers to an emergency when animal suffers severe hypoxia and carbon dioxide accumulation. The main phenotypes include cyanosis, extreme breathing difficulty, and breathing slowing down. Most of the experimental animal asphyxia is caused by respiratory tract obstruction. If asphyxia is treated in time, it will not result in serious consequences. Otherwise the experimental animal will die. In chronic animal experiments, no tracheal intubation is needed; the animal will have difficulty of breath or even asphyxia because of relaxing of pharyngeal muscles after anesthesia. Pull out the tongue of the animal and fix it to one side to relieve asphyxia. In acute animal experiments, tracheal cannula with an inclined plane at the end may cause airway obstruction when the plane is attached to the tracheal wall. Rotate the cannula 180 degrees. When the airway is obstructed by tracheal secretions (accompany by stridor) or blood clots (without stridor), pull out the tracheal cannula, clean the cannula and trachea, and do tracheal intubation again.

2.5.7   Killing the Experimental Animal

At the end of the experiment, the animal should be killed. The principle is making the animal die quickly and painlessly.

Rabbits are usually killed by air embolism method, which involves using a syringe to inject a large amount of air into the vein or heart, causing widespread air embolism. The rabbits will die immediately. Rats and mice were usually killed by cervical vertebra dislocation. This method involves using the left thumb and forefinger to hold the animal head, using the right hand to hold the tail or body, pull forcefully to make the cervical vertebra dislocate.

The dead animal should be placed in the specified location for centralized processing.

(Tong Zan)

Chapter 3   Cellular Physiology

Experiment 1   The Frog Sciatic Nerve-Gastrocnemius Muscle Preparation

[**Purpose**]

To study the basic dissection and make a Sciatic nerve-Gastrocnemius muscle Preparation with excitability.

[**Principle**]

Preparing a frog nerve-muscle sample is a basic technique in a physiology experiment. Some of frogs' basic life activities are similar to that of homothermal animal. The sciatic nerve-gastrocnemius muscle preparation is functional in vitro, and this can be prolonged for several hours when it is incubated in Ringer's solution. Therefore, it is used to investigate the physiology of skeletal muscle and nerve, as well as the stimulation and responses of skeletal muscle.

[**Objects**]

toad or frog.

[**Materials and Equipments**]

Ringer's solution, Dissecting kit (including dissecting board, glass board, pithing needle, rough scissors, surgical scissors, fine scissors, glass rods, thread, beaker).

[**Experimental Procedure**]

(1) Kill frog by a double pith. The frog will be killed by using a pith needle to destroy both the brain and the spinal cord (double pithed).

Hold the frog in one hand, use the index finger to bend the head slightly downward, and insert the pith needle into the foramen (the slight depression between the skull and spinal cord). Move the needle to a position parallel to the top of the skull, push the point forward into the brain, and move the point from side to side to destroy the brain. Then reverse the direction of the pin and run the needle down the spinal cord to destroy the cord. When this double pith is complete, the hind legs will become extended and then will relax.

(2) Sever the spinal cord below the skull and remove the abdominal organs. Cut the skin along the spinal column to rump bone. Cut through the abdominal musculature and carefully

remove the abdominal organs. This exposes the three roots of the sciatic nerve on either side of the vertebral column.

(3) Remove the skin carefully. Hold the vertebral column (be careful not to touch the sciatic nerve on both sides) with one hand, catch the skin and remove it with another hand. Put the preparation without skin into Ringer's solution. Clear up all instruments used.

(4) Separate the two legs. Lay the preparation on a clean glass plate. Separate the two legs by cutting through the median line. Put one half in Ringer's solution for backup preparation, and use the other half for further dissection.

(5) Dissect the sciatic nerve from the surrounding muscles in the thigh using a glass rod. Fix the preparation on dissection board with upward motion. Starting at the spinal end, insert a thread under all nerves and tie them, leaving enough thread to hang onto. Now cut the central part of nerves, carefully lift it by the thread. With fine scissors, free the sciatic nerve from connective tissue as it runs peripherally. Continue isolating the nerve from the upper leg until it reaches the knee. Cut away the muscles from the femur, leaving the nerve exposed, and with a section of the femur left (about 2-3 cm) to anchor the preparation in subsequent experiments.

(6) Just above the heel, insert a scissor blade under the tendon and rotate it slightly to loosen the tendon. Pass a moistened thread around the Achilles tendon at the heel and tie it tightly around the tendon. Lift the tendon with forceps, and with scissors, cut the fascia binding the gastrocnemius to the neighboring structures. Cut away the tibia and the fibula just below the knee. Tie a thread just above the belly of the tendon. The preparation is now completed. Keep the preparation moist in the Ringer's solution.

(7) Examine the excitability of nerve-muscle preparation using Zinc-Copper probe.

[Observations]

Test the excitability of the preparation. Put the preparation on glass plate, lift up the sciatic nerve, and create a shock using a Zinc-Copper probe soaked in Ringer's solution. The excitability of the preparation is good if the gastrocnemius muscle makes a quick and strong contraction.

[Notices]

(1) Toads can squirt a spray of secretion when they are handled for destroying the brain and spinal cord. When the eyes have been exposed to toad secretion, wash with a lot of water and saline.

(2) Keep the preparation moist with Ringer's solution at all times.

(3) Do not touch the nerve with any metal point or fingers unless specifically instructed to do so. Handle with glass hook only.

[Questions]

1. How to determine whether the toad's brain and spinal cord are destroyed completely?

2. How does the zinc-copper probe check the excitability of the sciatic nerve-gastrocnemius muscle preparation?

[**Key Words**]

   sciatic nerve-gastrocnemius muscle   excitability

(Zhang Xianrong)

Experiment 2   Effect of the Stimulation Intensity on Skeletal Muscle Contraction

[**Purpose**]

   (1) Describe the effect of stimulus intensity on muscle contraction strength.

   (2) Demonstrate the recruitment of motor units with increasing strength of stimuli to the motor nerve.

[**Principle**]

   Muscular, nervous, and glandular tissues are referred to as excitable tissues. They are capable of producing electrical signals when stimulated. In the nerve, this electric impulse can be conducted along the trunk. In muscular tissues, this electric phenomenon is associated with the contraction through excitation-contraction coupling. Generally, the minimal stimulation intensity required for excitation of cells is used to evaluate the excitability of the cells. Stimulation can be characterized by three parameters including stimulation intensity, stimulation duration, and intensity-time ramp. In physiological experiments, square pulses are always used for stimulation. When the stimulation duration is set to a constant level, the minimal stimulation intensity which can excite the tissue is called threshold intensity (or threshold stimulation), and the minimal stimulation intensity which can induce the maximum response is called the maximum stimulation.

[**Objects**]

   toad or frog.

[**Materials and Equipments**]

   Pithing needle, glass rod, glass plate, rough scissors, surgical scissors, fine scissors, Ringer's solution, thread, beaker, Muscle chamber, tension transducer, RM6240 physiological recording system.

[**Experimental Procedure**]

   (1) In vitro Sciatic nerve-Gastrocnemius muscle preparation.

   (2) Fix the preparation in the nerve/muscle chamber. Place the sciatic nerve on the wire electrodes in the nerve/muscle chamber, and attach the femur to the bone clamp. Secure the thread attached to the lower end of the gastrocnemius to the tension transducer.

   (3) Equipment setup. Connect tension transducer leads to the Channel 1 input on the pedestal. Connect the stimulator output cable to the stimulation electrode on nerve/muscle chamber(Figure 3-1).

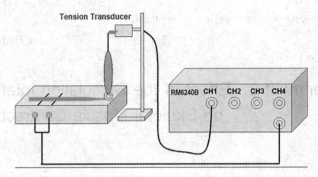

Figure 3-1   The setup to record excitation-contraction from sciatic nerve-gastrocnemius muscle

[Observations]

(1) Select appropriate program in the "experiment" menu. Click on the "stimulator" icon to open the dialog box, set stimulation mode as single, square wave voltage of positive stimulation with wave-width 0. 2-0. 5 ms. Increase the stimulus intensity in steps of appropriate stimulus voltage. Start stimulation, recording the changes of muscle contraction in response to increasing stimulation intensity.

(2) The stimulator voltage will be gradually increased from zero to an intensity where a muscle twitch first appears, this minimal stimulus voltage is called threshold stimulus. The contraction amplitudes will increase along with increasing stimulation intensity. When the contraction amplitudes reach a maximum amplitude and keep in a constant level regardless of increasing stimulation intensity, the minimal stimulation intensity which induces the maximum response (the contraction amplitude reaches the maximum) is called maximum stimulus intensity(Figure 3-2).

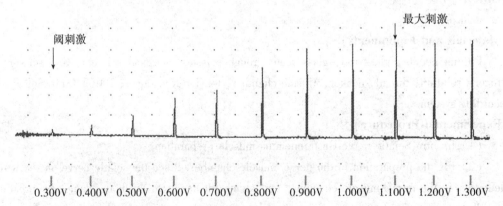

Figure 3-2   The effect of stimulation intensity on gastrocnemius muscle contraction

[**Notices**]

(1) To maintain the excitability and contractibility of nerve-muscle sample in agood state, let the preparation stay for 0. 5-1 min after each stimulation.

(2) Keep the preparation moist with Ringer's solution at all times.

[**Questions**]

1. What's the change of muscle contraction amplitude in response to increasing stimulation intensity? What's the underlying mechanism?

2. How does the stimulation on sciatic nerve induce the contraction of gastrocnemius muscle?

[**Key Words**]

threshold stimulus	threshold intensity
minimal stimulus	maximal stimulus
excitation	excitability

(Zhang Xianrong)

Experiment 3   Effect of the Frequency of Stimulus on Skeletal Muscle Contraction

[**Object**]

To record the effect of stimulus frequency on skeletal muscle contraction and demonstrate three types of contraction: single twitch, incomplete tetanus, and complete tetanus.

[**Introduction**]

Skeletal muscle is innervated by motor nerves. Stimulation on the nerve trunk excites nerve fibers, then the electrical pulse can be conducted along the nerve fibers, and in turn cause activation of muscle cells through the neuromuscular junctions. The frequency of electrical pulses conducted along nerve fibers affect the form and strength of muscle contraction. In this experiment, the strength of stimulus is held constant and only the frequency of stimulus is increased. When the stimuli are applied at a frequency where the time interval between stimuli is longer than the time it takes for the muscle fibers to completely contract and relax, then no tetanus is observed, the contraction is called single twitch. When the stimuli is applied at a frequency where the time interval between stimuli is shorter than the time it takes for the muscle fibers to completely relax, then incomplete tetanus is observed. If the stimuli are applied at a frequency where the time interval is shorter than the time it takes for the muscle fibers to even begin to relax, then complete tetanus is observed.

[**Objects**]

toad or frog.

[**Materials and Equipments**]

pithing needle, glass rod, glass plate, heavy scissors, fine scissors, Ringer's solution, thread, beaker, Nerve/Muscle chamber, tension transducer, RM6240 physiological recording system.

[**Experimental Procedure**]

(1) Prepare the Sciatic nerve-Gastrocnemius muscle Preparation.

(2) Fix the preparation in the nerve/muscle chamber. Place the sciatic nerve on the wire electrodes in the nerve/muscle chamber, and attach the femur to the bone clamp. Secure the thread attached to the lower end of the gastrocnemius to the tension transducer.

(3) Equipment setup. Connect the tension transducer leads to the Channel 1 input on the pedestal. Connect the stimulator output cable to the stimulation electrode on nerve/muscle chamber.

[**Observations**]

Select appropriate program in the "experiment" menu. Set up stimulation parameters: Adjust the stimulator so that the stimulus strength is enough to produce a good twitch. Hold the strength of stimulus constant and only increase the frequency of stimulus. Other parameters are set as following:

Single twitch, stimulus frequency: 1Hz, pulse number: 1;

Incomplete tetanus: stimulus frequency: 8-16 Hz, pulse number: 5-15;

Complete tetanus: stimulus frequency: 25-40Hz, pulse number: 10-25.

Effect of different frequency o stimulus on skeletal muscle contraction is shown in Figure 3-3.

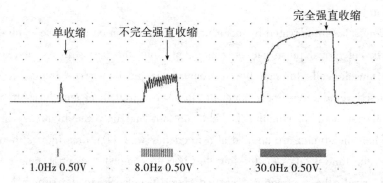

Figure 3-3   single twitch, incomplete tetanus and complete tetanus of
skeletal muscle in response to different frequency of stimulus

[**Notices**]

(1) To maintain the excitability and contractibility of the nerve-muscle sample in a good state, let the preparation stay for 0.5-1 min after each stimulation.

(2) Keep the preparation moist with Ringer's solution at all times.

[**Questions**]

1. When the skeletal muscle contracts, are the amplitudes of contraction the same among single twitch, incomplete tetanus, and complete tetanus?

2. What is the difference between skeletal contraction and cardiac muscle contraction?

[**Key Words**]

　　single twitch　　　incomplete tetanus　　　complete tetanus

(Zhang Xianrong)

Experiment 4　Compound Action Potential in the Frog's Sciatic Nerve

[**Purpose**]

(1) To record the compound action potentials in the toad sciatic nerve.

(2) To determine the amplitude, latent period, duration, and wave form of the compound action potentials.

[**Principle**]

When the stimulating voltage reaches a sufficient level (the threshold), the region of the nerve beneath the stimulating electrodes becomes depolarized (the outside of the nerve becomes negative with respect to the inside). The action potential will be generated once the depolarization reaches the threshold potential and it is then conducted from the stimulating electrodes toward the recording electrodes. The positive and negative phases of the action potential are then recorded with a pair of extracellular electrodes, and is called biphasic action potential. When the nerve is damaged between these two electrodes, this action potential reaches the first recording electrode, but will not reach the region of the second electrode. It becomes electrically negative with respect to the second electrode, and monophasic action potential is recorded.

The frog's sciatic nerves are composed of bundles of thousands of individual nerve fibers which are enclosed in a connective tissue sheath. Therefore, the compound action potential is different from action potential recorded from a single nerve fiber. The compound action potentials are the summation of many individual "all-or-none" action potentials generated almost simultaneously in a large number of individual nerve fibers. The amplitudes of compound action potential will change with the alteration of stimulin a certain range of intensities.

[**Objects**]

　　toad or frog.

[**Materials and Equipments**]

　　Dissection kit (pithing needle, glass rod, glass plate, heavy scissors, fine scissors),

Ringer's solution, thread, beaker, Nerve/Muscle chamber, tension transducer, RM6240 physiological recording system.

[**Experimental Procedure**]

(1) Sciatic nerve preparation   Kill a frog by double pith. The surgical procedure is similar to that of making a sciatic nerve-gastrocnemius muscle preparation. Dissect the sciatic nerve from the surrounding muscles in the thigh using a glass rod. Starting at the spinal end, insert a thread under all the nerves and tie them, leaving enough thread to hang onto. Now cut the central part of the nerves and begin to carefully lift by the thread, and with fine scissors cut the sciatic free from connective tissue as it runs peripherally. Cut the branches divergent from the main nerve. Continue isolating the nerve from the upper leg until it reaches the knee. Here tie another ligature, then cut the nerve beyond this point and lift it free from the body. Immerse it in a beaker of Ringer's solution for further experimentation.

(2) Instrument setup   Hold the thread on both ends of the nerve, lay the nerve across the stimulating and two sets of recording electrodes in the nerve chamber, and cover the chamber with the lid(Figure 3-4). Connect the output stimulating leads with the stimulating electrodes in the nerve chamber, and connect the recording electrodes to the leads which inputs the signals to Channel 1.

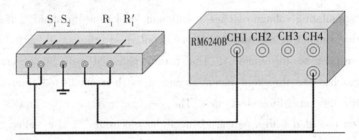

Figure 3-4   The setup to record compound action potential on sciatic nerve

(3) Parameter setup Select experiment program, set up parameters as following: select "synchronizer trigger", positive voltage stimulation mode, single stimulus with intensity: 0. 1-1v, pulse width: 0. 1-0. 2ms.

[**Observations**]

(1) The relationship between the amplitude of compound action potential and stimulation intensity. Increase of stimulation intensity in a certain range causes the amplitude of compound action potential to increase simultaneously. Record the threshold intensity and maximal stimulation intensity with a certain pulse width.

(2) Biphasic action potential. Record the latent period, maximal peak amplitude, and duration of biphasic compound action potential induced by maximal stimulus.

(3) Monophasic action potential. Use forceps to damage the nerve or block nerve conduction by drug (procaine) between two recording electrodes. Stimulate the nerve, and if

the second phase of the biphasic action potential is absent, the potential recorded is monophasic action potential. Record the latent period, maximal peak amplitude, and duration of monophasic compound action potential induced by maximal stimulus.

Biphasic and monophasic action potential in frog's sciatic nerve is shown in Figure 3-5.

(Zhang Xianrong)

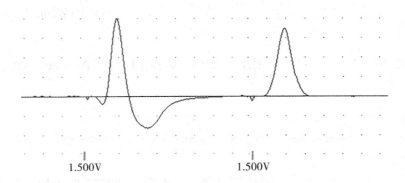

1.500V   1.500V

Figure 3-5 Biphasic action potential and monophasic action potential

[**Notices**]

(1) Be careful not to damage the nerve during surgical procedure. When handling the sample, hold the threads using forceps on both ends of the nerve sample, don't clip directly on the nerve.

(2) Keep the preparation moist with Ringer's solution at all times. Care should be taken to avoid short circuit induced by excessive Ringer's solution between electrodes.

(3) The nerve preparation should be placed straight on electrodes in good contact.

(4) The proximal end of the nerve (that end connected to the spinal column) should be over the stimulating electrodes, and the distal end (from the knee region) should be over the recording electrodes. The threads on both ends of the nerve sample should not be in contact with the wall of the nerve chamber.

(5) Stimulus should be administered in appropriate intensity, and stimulation should not be too frequent, otherwise too much stimulation will damage the nerve preparation.

[**Questions**]

1. Is there any change in the amplitude and wave form of compound action potential with increasing stimulus intensity? Please explain the underlying mechanism of this change.

2. Are the amplitude and wave form of the compound action potential the same as that recorded from a single neuron? Why?

3. Why are the positive phase and negative phase of the biphasic compound action potential not symmetrical?

4. Why is the compound action potential biphasic? Why does the compound action

potential become monophasic when the nerve between the two recording electrodes is damaged?

5. How is a stimulation artifact generated? How to identify the compound action potential from stimulation artifact? How to reduce or eliminate the stimulation artifact?

[**Key Words**]

action potential

monophasic action potential

biphasic action potential

compound action potential.

(Zhang Xianrong)

Experiment 5   The Conduction Velocity of Nerve Impulse

[**Purpose**]

To examine the conduction velocity of compound action potentials in the sciatic nerve.

[**Principle**]

When the sciatic nerve is excited by stimulation with appropriate intensity, the action potential will be conducted along the nerve fibers at a certain velocity. The conduction velocity varies in different types of nerve fibers. The thicker the nerve fiber, the faster the conduction velocity in the fiber. The majority of fibers in the frog's sciatic nerve are Aa; the conduction velocity in Aa fibers is around 30-40 m/s. Measure the distance of action potentials which are conducted on the nerve, and the time interval which the action potential conducted on this certain distance. Calculate the conduction velocity of the action potential on the nerve according to the formula $v=s/t$.

[**Objects**]

toad or frog.

[**Materials and Equipments**]

Dissection kit (pithing needle, glass rod, glass plate, heavy scissors, fine scissors), Ringer's solution, thread, beaker, Nerve/Muscle chamber, tension transducer, RM6240 physiological recording system.

[**Experimental Procedures**]

(1) Sciatic nerve preparation. Prepare sciatic nerve sample following the procedure in experiment 4.

(2) Instrument setup. Hold the thread on both ends of the nerve, lay the nerve across the stimulating and two sets of recording electrodes in the nerve chamber, and cover the chamber with the lid. Connect the output stimulating leads with the stimulating electrodes in the nerve chamber, and connect the recording electrodes to the leads which inputs the signals to Channels 1 and 2(Figure 3-6).

(3) Parameter setup. Select experiment program, set up parameters as following: select "synchronizer trigger" , positive voltage stimulation mode, single stimulus with intensity: 0. 1-

1v, pulse width: 0. 1-0. 2ms.

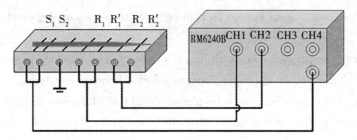

Figure 3-6   The setup to measure conduction velocity of compound action potential on the sciatic nerve.

[**Observations**]

(1) Measure the latent period of the compound action potential recorded from 2 pairs of recording electrodes (duration from stimulus artifact to the initiation point of compound action potential), represented by t_1 and t_2, respectively. The difference between t_2 and t_1 (t_2-t_1) is the duration (Δt) that the action potential will be conducted from R_1 to R_2. Generally, it is hard to identify the initial point of the action potential, therefore, we always use the duration of the peak wave of first phase between two compound action potentials to represent the duration (Δt).

(2) Measure the distance (s) between the first electrodes of two pairs of recording electrodes.

(3) Calculate the conduction velocity of compound action potentials using the following formula: $v=s/t$ (Figure 3-7).

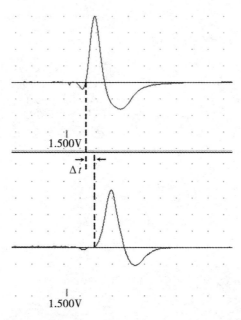

Figure 3-7   Determination of conduction velocity of compound action potentials on the sciatic nerve.

[**Notices**]

(1) Be careful not to damage the nerve during the surgical procedure. When handling the sample, hold the threads using forceps on both ends of the nerve sample, don't clip directly on the nerve.

(2) Keep the preparation moist with Ringer's solution at all times. Care should be taken to avoid short circuit induced by excessive Ringer's solution between electrodes.

(3) The nerve preparation should be placed straight on electrodes in good contact.

(4) The proximal end of the nerve (that end connected to the spinal column) should be over the stimulating electrodes, and the distal end (from the knee region) should be over the recording electrodes. The threads on both ends of nerve sample should not be in contact with the wall of the nerve chamber.

(5) Stimuli should be administered in appropriate intensities, and stimulation should not be too frequent, otherwise too much stimulation will damage the nerve preparation.

[**Questions**]

1. Is there any difference regarding the amplitude, duration, and wave form between the compound action potential recorded from two pairs of recording electrodes? What's the underlying mechanism of this difference?

2. Please describe those impact factors which affect the conduction velocity of action potentials on nerve fibers.

[**Key Words**]

action potential   conduction velocity   compound action potential

(Zhang Xianrong)

Chapter 4   Blood

Experiment 6   Osmotic Fragility Test of Erythrocytes

[**Purpose**]

(1) To study the method of osmotic fragility test of erythrocytes.

(2) To observe the morphological change of erythrocytes in sodium chloride solution with varied concentrations.

[**Principle**]

Osmosis depends on the passive diffusion of water across a membrane from a region of low solute concentration to a region of high solute concentration. **Osmolality** is defined as the total number of dissolved particles per kg of solvent, and has units of mOsmol/kg. **Osmotic pressure** is the hydrostatic pressure that would be necessary to exactly oppose the osmotic effect of a solution and prevent any net water movement. **Isoosmotic solution** is in osmotic equilibrium with the osmotically active solutes in intracellular fluid under normal conditions. **Hyperosmotic solution** contains a higher concentration of osmotically active particles than the intracellular fluid, leading to osmotic water loss and cell shrinking. **Hypoosmotic solution** contains a lower concentration of osmotically active particles than the intracellular fluid, leading to osmotic cell swelling and possibly cell lysis. 0.9% NaCl is not only isosmotic but also isotonic. When erythrocytes are suspended in 0.9% NaCl, the amount of water diffusing in the two directions through the cell membrane is balanced so that the normal shape and size of erythrocytes are maintained. When erythrocytes are suspended in graded hypotonic solutions, net movement of water occurs from the bathing solution into cell, leading to cell swelling and even hemolysis. The osmotic resistance of erythrocyte to hypotonic solution is described by concentration of hypotonic NaCl solution that induces hemolysis. The concentration of NaCl that initiates hemolysis is called **maximal fragility**, and the concentration of NaCl that induces all of the erythrocytes to hemolyze is called **minimal fragility**.

[**Object**]

Rabbit.

[**Materials and Equipments**]

(1) Equipment: operating instruments of mammalian, artery clip, operating table of

rabbit, artery cannula, syringe (1 ml), tubes.

(2) Solutions and drugs: 20% ethyl carbamate, 1% NaCl, distilled water.

[**Experimental Procedures**]

1. Preparations of Graded Hypotonic Solution

Make a series of dilution to the stock solution of 1% NaCl in 10 tubes(Table 4-1).

Table 4-1

Tube No.	1	2	3	4	5	6	7	8	9	10
1%NaCl(ml)	1.80	1.40	1.20	1.10	1.00	0.90	0.80	0.70	0.60	0.50
H_2O (ml)	0.20	0.60	0.80	0.90	1.00	1.10	1.20	1.30	1.40	1.50
NaCl(%)	0.90	0.70	0.60	0.55	0.50	0.45	0.40	0.35	0.30	0.25

2. Anesthesia and Fixation

20% ethyl carbamate (dose: 5ml/kg body weight) is injected into the marginal ear vein. After the disappearance of the corneal reflex, fix the rabbit on the operating table and turn on the light at the table bottom to maintain temperature.

3. Artery Intubation

Shear the hair on the neck, cut open skin along the middle cervical line, and separate the trachea with hemostats. Pull apart the skin and muscles above the trachea with hemostats, and separate the right or left common carotid artery and insert the artery cannula.

4. Observation Items

Loosen the arterial clip slowly, add a few drops of blood into the tubes, and gently mix. After standing for 1 hour, observe the change of the mixture in the tube.

(1) If the mixture separates into a lower red, turbid phase, and an upper colorless, clear phase, hemolysis does not occur.

(2) If the mixture separates into a lower red, turbid phase, and an upper red, clear phase, a part of the red blood cells are hemolyzed.

(3) If the mixture presents red, clear phase, all of the red blood cells are hemolyzed.

[**Notices**]

(1) Carefully separate blood vessels to prevent from injuring them.

(2) Stop bleeding immediately whenever it takes place in operation.

(3) The amount of blood added into each tube should be consistent.

(4) After adding blood into the tubes, gently mix the solution.

[**Questions**]

How to analyze the minimal fragility and maximal fragility?

[**Key Words**]

osmotic pressure   isoosmotic solution

(Li Changyong)

Experiment 7　Blood Types and Cross Matching

[Purpose]

(1) To study the method of blood typing.

(2) To understand the cross matching in Clinic.

[Principle]

Whenever antigens on the surface of erythrocytes (**agglutinogens**) come into contact with specific antibodies directed against them (**agglutinins**), the cells clump together or agglutinate. By testing for agglutination of erythrocytes with known antibodies, the erythrocyte antigens can be identified and this defines the **blood group**. There are two main antigens, A and B, and these give rise to four different blood groups as shown in Table 4-2.

Table 4-2

Genotype	Antigens on cells	Antibodies in plasma	Blood group
OO	None	Anti-A and anti-B	O
OA or AA	A	Anti-B	A
OB or BB	B	Anti-A	B
AB	A and B	None	AB

Donor and recipient blood groups should normally match. Donor cells are mixed with recipient plasma, while recipient cells are mixed with donor plasma; there should be no agglutination in either case. This is referred to as **cross matching**.

[Object]

Human.

[Materials and Equipments]

(1) Equipment: blood taking needle, biconcave slide.

(2) Solutions and drugs: physiological saline, 75% ethanol, standard serum A, standard serum B.

[Experimental Procedures]

Prepare standard serum A and B on biconcave slide, and then add one drop of blood in standard serum A and B, respectively.

[Notices]

(1) The position of blood collection should be sterilized with 75% ethanol.

(2) Avoid the mixture of standard serum A and B on biconcave slide.

[Questions]

What is the mechanism of identification of the different blood groups?

[Key Words]

agglutinogens   blood type

(Li Changyong)

Experiment 8   Blood Coagulation and the Impact Factors

[Purpose]

To analyze the impact factors on blood coagulation.

[Principle]

There are two pathways involved in blood coagulation: **intrinsic system** in which all blood-clotting factors are present in plasma and **extrinsic system** in which the initiated activator (tissue factor) comes from the tissue but not blood. In the experiment, blood is directly removed from the artery without contact with tissue factor, so blood coagulation is initiated through an intrinsic pathway. In both the extrinsic and intrinsic pathways, a series of different plasma proteins called blood-clotting factors play a major role. Most of these proteins are inactive forms of proteolytic enzymes. When converted to the active forms, their enzymatic actions cause the successive, cascade reactions of the clotting process. Blood coagulation is a complicated proteolytic process, and is affected by many factors such as the temperature, the smoothness of contact surface, and some substance.

[Object]

Rabbit.

[Materials and Equipments]

(1) Equipment: operating instruments of mammalian, artery clip, operating table of rabbit, artery cannula, beakers.

(2) Solutions and drugs: 20% ethyl carbamate, 0.9% sodium chloride, heparin, potassium oxalate, liquid paraffin, cotton.

[Experimental Procedures]

1. Anesthesia and Fixation

20% ethyl carbamate (dose: 5ml/kg body weight) is injected into the marginal ear vein. After the disappearance of the corneal reflex, fix the rabbit on operating table, and turn on the light at the table bottom to maintain temperature.

2. Artery Intubation

Shear the hair on the neck, cut open skin along the middle cervical line, and separate the trachea with hemostats. Pull apart the skin and muscles above the trachea with hemostats, and separate the right or left common carotid artery and insert the artery cannula.

3. Observation Items

Loosen the arterial clip slowly, and add 10 ml of blood into each beaker under different conditions and mix gently, record the time. Check blood fluidity every 30s by leaning the beakers, and record time required for blood clotting in Table 4-3.

Table 4-3

Beaker No.	Treatment	Blood clotting time
1	Control	
2	Incubated at 37-40℃	
3	Incubated at 0℃	
4	Paved with a little cotton	
5	Lubricated by liquid paraffin	
6	Addition of heparin (8U)	
7	Addition of potassium oxalate (5mg)	
8	Continuous stir to remove the formed fibrin	

[**Notices**]

(1) Carefully separate blood vessels to prevent injuring them. Stop bleeding immediately whenever it takes place in operation.

(2) The amount of blood added into each tube should be the same.

(3) Record the blood clotting time from addition of blood into beakers to complete coagulation. During this period, check blood fluidity every 30s by leaning the beakers.

[**Questions**]

What are the mechanisms of the above factors influencing blood coagulation?

[**Key Words**]

coagulation

(Li Changyong)

Chapter 5　Circulation

Experiment 9　Analysis of Heart Pacemaker

[**Purpose**]

(1) To study the method of exposing the heart of the frog and to know the anatomy of heart;

(2) To observe the effect of local temperature on autorhythmicity of heart;

(3) To observe heart pacemaker and different autorhythmicity at specific parts of the heart by Straub's ligation.

[**Principle**]

The cardiac specific conduction system has automatic rhythmicity, whereas the autorhythmicity is different at specific parts of the heart. In mammals, the sinus node has the highest autorhythmicity. Normally, the excitation from sinus node can be conducted to atrium, ventricle and induce the contraction of them in turns. Based on the mechanism, the sinus node in mammals is also called the pacemaker of the heart. In amphibians, the venous sinus has the highest autorhythmicity, hence it is the pacemaker of the heart. In physiological conditions, the rhythmicity of a whole frog heart is controlled by venous sinus. The venous sinus, atrium, and ventricle contract in turns. When the conduction of excitation from normal pacemaker is blocked, the lower autorhythmicity from the other part of the heart could be observed.

[**Objects**]

Toad/frog.

[**Materials and Equipments**]

(1) Equipment: operating instruments of frog/toad, pins, frog heart clip, tube, thread.

(2) Solution: Ringer's solution, ice cold water and 37℃ water.

[**Experimental Procedures**]

1. Operation

Destroy brain and spinal cord of toad. Fix the four legs of the toad with pins on the operation board with the thoracic cavity side up (Figure 5-1). Hold the skin below the xiphoid and cut open the skin, cutting the skin from xiphoid to both collar bones to expose muscle at thoracic cavity. Cut off the muscle below the xiphoid to make a hole, cut open the thoracic cavity alongside the incision of skin. Cut off the collar bones and the coracoid of both sides. Turnover and transversely cut off the tissue to expose the thoracic cavity of the frog. Cut open the pericardium with fine scissors.

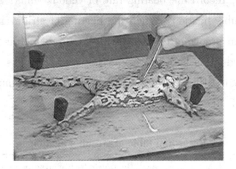

Figure 5-1   Fix the legs of the toad with the thoracic cavity side up.

2. Observe the Anatomy of Heart

From the ventral side, the atriums, ventricle and atrioventricular groove can be observed. The conus arteriosus is on the right side of ventricle, which is the swollen root of the aorta. The aorta goes up and separates into two branches (Figure 5-2). Turnover the heart with the glass needle and the venous sinus can be observed under the atriums. There is a white boundary line between atrium and venous sinus, which is called sinus sulcus.

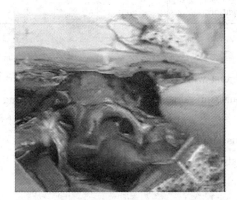

Figure 5-2   Heart photo from the ventral side of frog.

3. Observations

(1) Observe the normal heart beating: observe the order and rate of venous sinus, atrium, and ventricle.

(2) The impact of local temperature of heart on autorhythmicity of heart: touch venous sinus or ventricle with 37℃ water or ice cold water separately, observe and record heart beating rate.

(3) The first straub's ligation: ligate on the sinus sulcus of the heart with thread, which is named the first straub's ligation, to block the transduction between venous sinus and atrium. Observe the changes of beating rate at specific parts of the heart. When the beating of atrium and ventricle is recovered, record the beating rate of venous sinus, atrium, and ventricle.

(4) The second straub's ligation: When the beating of atrium and ventricle is recovered, ligate on the atrioventricular groove of the heart with thread, which is named the second straub's ligation, to block the transduction between atrium and ventricle. Observe the changes of beating rate of different parts of heart. Record the beating rate of venous sinus, atrium, and ventricle.

(5) Fill the results in the table 5-1.

Table 5-1　　　　　　　　**Recording table of straub's ligation**

Observation items	Beating rate (beating per min)			Is the beating rate equal? (Y/N)
	Venous sinus	atrium	ventricle	
normal				
Touch venous sinus with 37℃ water				
Touch ventricle with 37℃ water				
Touch venous sinus with ice cold water				
Touch ventricle with ice cold water				
The first straub's ligation				
The second straub's ligation				

[**Notices**]

(1) Keep the heart moist with Ringer's solution when the heart is exposed.

(2) Protect the venous sinus during operation to avoid stopping the heart beating.

[**Questions**]

1. How can the venous sinus become the pace maker?

2. How does the beating of the ventricle change when we ligate between atrium and ventricle?

[**Key Words**]

pacemaker

(Wang Yuan)

Experiment 10　Premature Systole and Compensatory Pause

[**Purpose**]

(1) Observe the reaction of the heart when artificially given stimulation at the different

periods of activity of the heart, to verify the characteristics of the changes of excitability after excitation;

(2) To know how to record the contraction curve of the heart *in vivo*.

[**Principle**]

After the ventricular myocytes are activated, the excitability will change periodically, which are effective refractory, relative refractory and supernormal periods. The effective refractory period is very long, which covers the whole systole period and early diastole period of the heart contraction curve. During this period, the heart cannot trigger another excitation and contraction. But after early diastole period and before the next sinus excitation arrives, the heart can trigger another contraction which is premature systole if there is an additional super threshold stimulation. This extra systole has it's own excitation period, if the next sinus excitation arrives during the effective refractory period of the extra systole, the sinus excitation will not trigger a contraction of ventricular myocytes until the other sinus excitation arrives. The missing sinus excitation will cause a longer diastole than normal, which is named compensatory pause.

[**Objects**]

Toad/frog.

[**Materials and Equipments**]

(1) Equipment: RM6240 biological signal recording system, operating instruments of frog/toad, frog heart clip, tension transducer, stimulator.

(2) Solution: Ringer's solution.

[**Experimental Procedures**]

1. Operation

Destroy the brain and spinal cord of the toad. Fix the four legs of the toad with pins on the operation board with the thoracic cavity side up. Open the thoracic cavity to expose the heart with operating scissors and forceps.

2. Connecting with System

Clasp the heart apex at the diastole period by heart clip with thread connected. The other end of the thread connects the tension transducer, which connects with recording channel I of the RM6240 biological signal recording system.

The stimulator connects with stimulus output channel and the needle electrodes of the stimulator touch the ventricles of the heart.

3. Observations

(1) Choose premature systole and compensatory pause as the experiment model, record normal contraction curve of the toad's heart.

(2) Choose single stimulus with the parameters of 1-5V in intension, 1ms in duration/bandwidth, give stimulus at the different time point of the systole period and early diastole period. Observe the change of contraction curve.

(3) Give stimulus at the different time point of the middle and late diastole period. Observe the change of contraction curve.

(4) When premature contraction occurs, observe if there is a compensatory pause behind.

[**Notices**]

(1) Keep the toad heart moist with Ringer's solution.

(2) Make sure the needle electrodes touch the surface of ventricles during both diastole and systole period.

(3) Keep the control curve before giving a stimulus; wait for at least three cardiac cycles between two stimuli.

[**Questions**]

1. Explain the recorded curves; analyze the mechanism of premature systole and compensatory pause.

2. What is the character and physiological meaning of the excitability change after excitation of cardiomyocytes?

3. When the bradycardia or tachycardia occurs, is it certain that the compensatory pause occurs after premature pause?

[**Key Words**]

premature systole　　compensatory pause

(Wang Yuan)

Experiment 11　Observation of Frog Electrocardiogram in Vivo and in Vitro

[**Purpose**]

(1) To learn the characteristics of electrocardiogram (ECG) and know the relationship of ECG and action potential of cardiomyocytes.

(2) To know the phenomenon of volume conductor.

[**Principle**]

ECG is a transthoracic interpretation of the electrical activity of the heart in real time captured and externally recorded by skin electrodes. Electrodes on different sides of the heart measure the activity of different parts of the heart muscle.

[**Objects**]

Toad/frog.

[**Materials and Equipments**]

(1) Equipment: RM6240 biological signal recording system, operating instruments of frog/toad, frog heart clip.

(2) Solution: Ringer's solution.

[Experimental Procedures]

1. Operation

Destroy the brain and spinal cord of the toad. Fix the four legs of the toad with pins on the operation board with the thoracic cavity side up. Open the thoracic cavity to expose the heart with operating scissors and forceps.

2. Record ECG with lead II

The three electrodes from channel I of the RM6240 biological signal recording system have three colors. The negative electrode in green connects onto the pin of the right arm of the toad, the positive electrode in red connects onto the pin of the left leg of the toad, and the ground electrode in black connects onto the pin of the right leg of the toad.

3. Observations

(1) Choose toad ECG as the experiment model and start recording the electrocardiogram figure, observing the normal ECG from lead II (Figure 5-3). Observe the shape and orientation of the p wave, QRS waves and T wave.

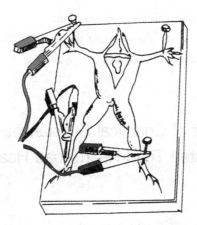

Figure 5-3   toad ECG connection with lead II.

(2) Turn over the heart with a glass needle to let the apex of the heart towards head, observing the changes of ECG on orientation and shape. Then turn the heart back and observe the changes of ECG.

(3) Cut and remove the toad heart from the thoracic cavity, observing the changes of ECG on orientation and shape.

(4) Return the heart back and observe the changes of ECG.

(5) Put the isolated heart into a dish with Ringer's solution, connect the three electrodes on the dish and let the position of the electrode be same as the orientation in the thoracic cavity (Figure 5-4). Observe characteristics of ECG.

(6) Change the direction of the electrodes on the dish and observe the changes of ECG.

(7) Remove the heart from the dish and observe the changes of ECG.

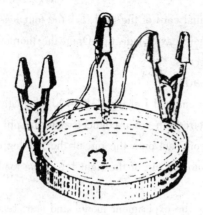

Figure 5-4   toad ECG connection from isolated heart.

[**Notices**]

    1. Keep the toad heart moist with Ringer's solution.

    2. Do not hurt the venous sinus when cutting the heart off from the thoracic cavity.

    3. Make sure the operation board and dish are insulated.

(Wang Yuan)

Experiment 12   Effect of Chemical Substances on the Activity of an Isolated Toad Heart -toad Heart Perfusion in Vitro

[**Purpose**]

    (1) To learn the method of isolated heart perfusion.

    (2) To observe the effects of several ion concentrations on heart activity.

[**Principle**]

Amphibian's hearts can keep rhythmic systole and diastole in vitro in Ringer's solution. Changing the concentration of some ions in perfusate, or adding some agonist or antagonist could impact the heart activity in vitro. The frog heart has 3 chambers: two atria and a single ventricle. The right atrium receives deoxygenated blood from various organs of the body. The left atrium receives oxygenated blood from the lungs and skin. Both atria empty blood into the single ventricle.

[**Object**]

    Toad/Frog.

[**Materials and Equipments**]

    (1) Equipment: RM6240 biological signal recording system, operating instruments of

frog/toad, frog heart clip, tension transducer, biconcave clamp, Strub frog heart cannula, beaker, thread, iron lining.

(2) Solutions: Ringer's solution, 0. 65% NaCl, 1% KCl, 2% $CaCl_2$, 3% lactid acid, 2. 5% $NaHCO_3$, 10^{-4} mol/L Adrenaline, 10^{-5} mol/L ACh.

[**Methods**]

1. Operation

(1) Pithing the toad: Destroy the brain and spinal cord by inserting the needle into the cranial cavity and the vertebral canal.

(2) Fixation of toad: Let the toad lie with the back on the toad board. Push the pins through the toad's hands and feet into the board.

(3) Preparation of heart: Fix the heart with the heart clip, across three pieces of thread under left aorta for fixation of straub's cannula, under the right aorta for blocking blood stream of right aorta, and under both of them for blocking the connecting tissues under venous sinus.

(4) Straub's intubation: Firstly, make an incision on the aorta, then insert the tip of the tube filled by Ringer's solution from the aorta into the ventricle (Figure 5-5 and Figure 5-6). Fix the tube and isolate the whole heart out of the body.

(5) Setup the equipment: Hold the thread of the heart clip and connect it to a tension transducer for signal recording.

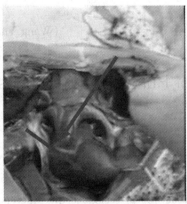

Figure 5-5   Insert orientation of the heart cannula intubation

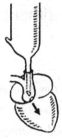

Figure 5-6   Heart cannula intubation model

2. Observations

(1) Record normal heart waves, mark the solution level on the cannula.

(2) Replace Ringer's solution with 0. 65% NaCl of same volume, observe changes of the heart beating. Wash out.

(3) Add 1-2 drops of 1% KCl, observe the change; wash out.

(4) Add 1 drop of 2% $CaCl_2$, observe the change; wash out.

(5) Add 1-2 drops of 3% lactic acid, observe the change of heart beating waves, then

add 2.5% $NaHCO_3$ of the same volume, wash out.

(6) Add 1-2 drops of 1 : 10 000 Adrenalin, observe the heart beating waves, wash out.

(7) Add 1-2 drops of 1 : 100 000 ACh, observe the heart beating waves, wash out.

[Notices]

(1) Keep the toad heart moist with Ringer's solution.

(2) Wash the straub's cannula at least three times with Ringer's solution after each observation item until the contraction waves are recovered.

(3) Make sure the perfusate amounts are equal between observations after washing.

(4) Do not mix different droppers for specific drugs.

[Questions]

1. How does the heart beating wave change when the perfusion Ringer's solution is taken place with 0.65% NaCl? Why?

2. How does the heart beating wave change when 1% KCl is added into perfusion Ringer's solution? Why?

3. How does the heart beating wave change when 3% $CaCl_2$ is added into perfusion Ringer's solution? Why?

4. How does the heart beating wave change when 1 : 10, 000 Adrenaline is added into perfusion Ringer's solution? Why?

5. How does the heart beating wave change when 1 : 100, 000 ACh is added into perfusion Ringer's solution? Why?

(Wang Yuan)

Experiment 13　Auscultation of Human Heart Sounds

[Purpose]

This experiment is based on the sound that human heart beats can be heard by stethoscope at the auscultation area of each valve in the chest during the cardiac cycle. The purpose is to learn the method of auscultation of human heart sounds and to recognize the difference of the first and second cardiac sounds, as well as to understand the characteristics of normal heart sounds and their mechanism.

[Experimental Principle]

The vibrations produced when the heart contracts and relaxes, valves open and close, blood rebounds against the ventricular walls or blood vessels in every cardiac cycle can pass through the surrounding tissues to the chest wall, which can conduct to the chest wall where the sound can be heard by stethoscope. The sound is called heart sound. There are four cardiac sounds in every cardiac cycle. But only the first and the second sounds can be heard in most normal human bodies. "The first cardiac sound": low-pitch and long duration. This sound is generated by the vibrations of the arterial wall and the closing of the atrioventricular valves which are caused by vortex blood hitting against expanded ventricular walls in ventricular ejection phase. It marks the beginning of systole because atrioventricular valves are closed while the systole begins. "The second cardiac sound": high-pitch and short duration. This sound is generated by the closing of the semilunar valves. It marks the beginning of diastole because the semilunar valves are closed while the diastole begins. The pitch reflects loudness of arterial pressure. Combination with cardiac impulse or carotid impulse can help the auscultation of heart sounds. The clinical sites of auscultation of heart sounds are as shown in the Figure 5-7.

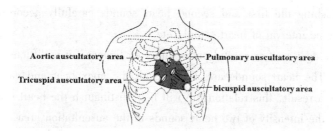

Figure 5-7   Diagram of heart sounds auscultation parts

[**Objects**]

Human beings.

[**Materials and Equipments**]

Stethoscope, stopwatch.

[**Experimental Procedures**]

1. Wearing a Stethoscope in the Correct Way

Stethoscope is made of the ear piece, the chest piece, and the rubber catheter components.

When you use the stethoscope, you should make the ear pieces directed to the same direction of the external auditory canal, and light hold stethoscope chest piece by your the right hand thumb, index finger, and middle finger.

2. Determining the Auscultation Sites

Subject is often in the position of supine or sitting, opening his or her jacket and facing a bright area. The examiner stands on the right side of the bed or sits opposite the subjects, finding the location and extent of subjects' apex beat through observation or palpation.

The auscultation areas of heart valves are divided to the four valves and five areas, as shown in Figure 5-7. ① the auscultation area of mitral valves: the fifth intercostal space slightly inside of the left mid-clavicular line (apex cordis); ② the auscultation area of tricuspid valves: the fourth intercostal space around the right edge of the sternum or xiphoid; ③ the auscultation area of aortic valve: the second intercostal space around the right edge of the sternum; ④ the second auscultation area of the aorta braid: the third intercostal space around the left edge of the sternum; ⑤ the auscultation area of the pulmonary valves: the second intercostal space around the left edge of the sternum.

3. Be familiar to the Order of Auscultation

This is generally heard according to the inverse of "8" stroke' auscultation areas, that is, the auscultation area of mitral valve → the auscultation area of aortic valve →the auscultation area of pulmonary valve →the auscultation area of tricuspid valve.

[**Experimental Item**]

1. Listen to heart sounds

(1) Distinguishing the first and second heart sounds carefully according loudness and pitch, duration, time interval of heart sound, etc.

(2)Touch the apex beat or carotid pulse with your fingers if it is difficult to distinguish the two heart sounds. The heart sounds are related with the apex beat and carotid pulse in the aspect of time, as a result, this relationship will help distinguish the heart sounds.

(3)Compare the intensity of two heart sounds in the auscultation area of valves.

(4)Judge whether the cardiac rhythm is neat or not.

2. Count the number of the heart rate (HR)

Place the chest piece of the stethoscope in the auscultation area of mitral valves, and then watch the number of the heart rate. If the rhythm is tidy, you can count the number of heart beats for only 15 seconds, which the four times is the heart rate.

[**Experimental Notices**]

(1)Keep the environment quiet and the examiner concentrated on the auscultation.

(2)Check if the piping system of the stethoscope is unblocked, and forbid silicone tube friction with other objects in order to avoid the influence of friction sound to auscultation.

(3)Ask the subjects to pause to breathe in case of breath sounds affecting the auscultation of heart sounds.

[**Questions**]

1. Is heart sound auscultation area in the appropriate anatomical location of each valve?

2. How to distinguish the first and second heart sounds?

3. Evaluation: which of the unusual activities can produce heart murmur or other abnormal heart sounds? As a result, it is significant to listen to heart sounds for the diagnosis of heart disease.

[**Key Words**]

cardiac sound　　　　auscultation

heart rate, HR　　　　cardiac rhythm

(Yan Xiaohong)

Experiment 14   Measurement of the Blood Pressure

[**Purpose**]

The blood pressure of human beings is measured by non-invasive, indirect convenient methods commonly used in clinical experiments. This is done by measuring blood pressure of the brachial artery in the upper arm to represent the individual's arterial pressure. The purpose of this experiment is to learn the method of measuring the arterial pressure in human being indirectly, and to measure the systolic pressure and diastolic pressure of the brachial artery.

[**Principle**]

The blood pressure is measured indirectly with a sphygmomanometer, and the most common way is the cuff auscultation according to the requisite pressure to suppress outside the artery by cuff of sphygmomanometer, which is also called as Korotkoff auscultation. Usually it is noiseless when the blood flows in blood vessels. But it sounds when the blood flows through a narrow place and a vortex current is formed. When air is filled into the rubbery cuff tied on the upper arm, its pressure exceeds to the systolic pressure and blocks the blood flow in the humeral artery completely. At this moment, no sound could be heard from the stethoscope with its chest piece placed on the terminal of the humeral artery and the pulse of the radial artery also could not be touched. When the pressure is lower than systolic pressure of the humeral artery and higher than diastolic pressure, the blood will flow interruptedly through the pressed blood vessels, form an eddy current, and produce sound. At this moment, sound could be heard from the stethoscope at the distal of the humeral artery and the pulse of the radial artery could be touched when the indication is the systolic pressure. Continuously discharge the gas till the outside pressure approximates to the diastolic pressure, the blood flow in the humeral artery will become more continuous as the blood flow increases, and the sound will be strong and clear. When the outside pressure equals to or is less than the diastolic pressure slightly, the blood flow in the humeral artery will become continuous from intermittent, and the sound will weaken or disappear. Then the pulse recovers to normal when the pressure in the cuff is diastolic pressure.

[**Object**]

Human beings.

[**Materials and Equipments**]

Stethoscope, sphygmomanometer, stopwatch.

[**Experimental Procedures**]

1. Knowing the Structure of Sphygmomanometer

Currently there are three kinds of sphygmomanometers, namely mercury column, clock-head style, and electronic sphygmomanometer. The sphygmomanometer is mainly made of the manometer, cuff, and a rubber ball (except for electronic sphygmomanometer). And the mercury manometer is a graduated glass tube with 0-260 mm, whose top is communicating with the atmosphere and bottom of groove of mercury. A clock-head style pressure gauge is seized with a pointer and scale of the dial and the pressure can push the pointer on the dial to rotate to a certain scale. The Cuff is an outsourcing rubber bag covered by the rectangular cloth which is respectively communicating with a mercury manometer and a rubber ball by rubber tubing. Rubber ball is a helical rubber bag with a ball valve, which is used for inflating and deflating. Electronic sphygmomanometer is made of an e-dial and electronic sphygmomanometer cuff, which can control automatically inflating, deflating, and display blood pressure values by the switch on electronic dial.

2. Method of Indirect Measurement of Arterial Blood Pressure

The subjects, in the general sitting or supine position, should make the midpoint of the upper arm and the heart on the same horizontal position when measured. Examiners touch arterial pulse through palpation to locate the brachial artery, and enwind the cuff on the forearm with proper tightness. The nether border of cuff should be 2-3 cm above the elbow joint at least. Membrane-type stethoscope chest piece is placed on the elbow fossa, where pulses of brachial arteries beat inside biceps. When air is filled into the rubbery cuff tied on the upper arm, its pressure exceeds to the systolic pressure and blocks the blood flow in the humeral artery completely. At this moment, no sound could be heard from the stethoscope. Continue to fill the air into the cuff until the mercury column increases by 20-30mmHg. Afterwards, deflating at the rate of 2-3 mmHg, when the pressure is lower than systolic pressure slightly, the blood will flow interruptedly through the pressed blood vessels from eddy current and produce sound. At this moment, the first sound (Korotkoff sound) could be heard from the stethoscope when the indication is the systolic pressure. When the pressure of the cuff equal to or slightly lower than the diastolic pressure, the blood flow completely restores and auscultation sounds disappear, and the indication is the diastolic pressure.

3. The Way of Blood Pressure Writing

often indicated by systolic / diastolic mmHg.

4. The Preparation before Measurement

(1) The subject calmly sits down for 5 to 10 minutes at first, and then takes off the sleeve of upper limb (usually the right upper limb). The subject is in the position of supine or sitting, keeping the height of forearm equal to the position of heart, arm straight, and mild outreach (Figure 5-8).

(2) Loosen the nut of the rubber ball, and lustrate the remaining gas from the cuff, and then fasten the nut.

(3) Align the cuff balloon portion of the brachial artery, and wind the cuff on the upper arm with proper tightness. The nether border of cuff should be 2-3 cm above the elbow joint at least.

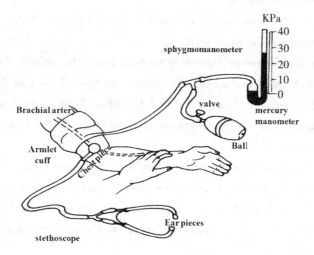

Figure 5-8   Schematic diagram of human arterial blood pressure measurement

(4) Check the person wearing a stethoscope, and first touch the pulse point of the humeral artery in the elbow fossa, and then put the chest piece of the stethoscope there, pressing it tight to contact the skin closely.

[**Experimental Item**]

(1) Measurement of the systolic pressure: use the rubber ball to pump gas into the rubber cuff to increase the pressure along with auscultation till the pulse of the humeral artery disappeared, and continue to pump gas to make the mercury column in the glass tube rises gradually near to 180mmHg. Whereat loosen the ball valve in the balloon, and deflate the gas slowly, keeping the eyes equal to the level of mercury column, as well as carefully listening to the sound. When hearing the first sound of pulse, pay attention to the height of the mercury column. The scale beside the height expresses the systolic pressure.

(2) Measurement of the diastolic pressure: continue deflating the gas slowly. The sounds are becoming increasingly strong as the mercury column decreases. And then there occurs a series of windy murmur sounds, and soon afterwards sounds become weak and low suddenly and at last disappears completely when the scale of mercury column represents the diastolic pressure.

[**Notices**]

(1) Keep the classroom silent to help auscultation.

(2) The cuff should be winded 2-3 cm above than the elbow band at least, and then the chest piece of the stethoscope should be put in the pulse point of the humeral artery and not under the cuff. The tightness of the cuff winded should be proper, neither loose nor tight.

(3) Arterial blood pressure can be measured twice continuously but should have an interval of 3-5 min. Besides, the pressure of the cuff must return to zero before the arterial

blood pressure is measured again.

(4) The position of the measurement is at the same level of the heart. Besides, the upper arm and the right atrium is the same level.

(5) When the blood pressure exceeds the normal scope, the subject should have a rest for 10 minutes and then be measured again. The subject can take off the cuff during the rest time.

(6) There are slight differences about 0.7-1.3 kPa (5-10 mmHg) between pressure of the left and righthumeral arteries. So sphygmomanometer should be fixed on one side and cannot be changed when measured.

(7) Use the sphygmomanometer in the proper way. Switch on the mercury chamber before pumping gas. After the experiment is over, lustrate the remaining gas from the cuff roll up the cuff and place it in the box. Place the manometer sphygmomanometer biasing to the right slightly and make the mercury return to the chamber of mercury, and then close the switch to avoid the mercury leaking.

[**Questions**]

1. What is systolic and diastolic blood pressure? How much is its normal value?

2. Explain the principle of systolic and diastolic measurement.

3. Why should the stethoscope chest piece not be placed under the cuff when the blood pressure is measured?

4. Why in a short time the measurement of arterial blood pressure cannot be measured repeatedly?

5. Evaluation: comparing arterial systolic and diastolic pressure measured by Korotkoff sound auscultation with that by the direct measurement method, the difference is less than 10%.

[**Key Words**]

arterial blood pressure   brachial artery

systolic pressure   diasystolic pressure

(Yan Xiaohong)

Experiment 15   Neural and Humoral Regulation of Circulatory System

[**Purpose**]

(1) Learn the method of recording the arterial blood pressure directly.

(2) Understand the effects of neural and humoral factors on cardiovascular activity.

[**Principle**]

The mammalian blood pressure maintains relatively stable under normal physiological conditions. This relative stability is achieved by the regulation of neural and humoral factors. In the neural regulation, the aortic arch baroreceptor reflex is particularly important, which can buck in the case of elevated blood pressure and boost when blood pressure is lowered. Afferent nerves in the reflex are aortic nerve and the carotid sinus nerve. The aortic nerve in the rabbit remains an independent tract and known as the depressor nerve, which is easy to be separated and checked. Efferent nerves in the reflex are the cardiac sympathetic nerve, cardiac vagus nerve and sympathetic vasoconstrictor nerve fiber. The cardiac sympathetic nerve releases norepinephrine when excited, and norepinephrine binds the β receptor on myocardial cell membrane resulting in the positive chronotropic, inotropic, and dromotropic effects on the heart. The cardiac vagus nerve releases acetylcholine when excited, and acetylcholine binds the M receptor on myocardial cell membrane resulting in negative chronotropic, inotropic, and dromotropic effects on the heart. The sympathetic vasoconstrictor fiber releases norepinephrine when excited, and norepinephrine binds the α receptor on vascular smooth muscle cell membrane resulting in increased peripheral resistance.

[**Objects**]

Rabbit.

[**Materials and Equipments**]

20% ethyl carbamate, heparin, 1 : 10 000 noradrenaline, 1 : 100 000 acetycholine, atropine, saline.

RM6240 physiological signal acquisition and processing system, operating instruments for mammals, tracheal cannula, blood pressure transducer, arterial cannula, artery clip, stimulating electrode, injectors, glass needle, gauze, fixing frames, thread.

[**Method and Procedures**]

(1) Anesthesia and fixation of the animal: Inject 20% ethyl carbamate into the ear vein slowly with the dose of 5 ml/kg, and fix the rabbit with its dorsal side down on the operating table.

(2) Prepare arterial cannula: Fill the blood pressure transducer and the arterial cannula with normal saline that contains 0.5% heparin through three-limb tube. Eliminate the air bubble in the blood pressure transducer and the arterial cannula.

(3) Separate cervical nerves and artery: shear the fur in the front of the neck; incise the cervical skin 6-8 cm along the midline carefully. Separate the muscles in the front of the thorax and separate the trachea. Clamp the edge of the incision with hemostatic forceps; lift and turn outside the cervical tissue beside the trachea using the index finger of the other hand, exposing the vascular plexus. The depressor nerve is the thinnest nerve compared to the vagus and sympathetic nerve (Figure 5-9). Use a glass needle to separate the vagus and depressor nerve 2 cm carefully, and put a saline moistened thread under the nerve. Use a glass needle to separate the common carotid artery and put two saline moistened threads under the vessel.

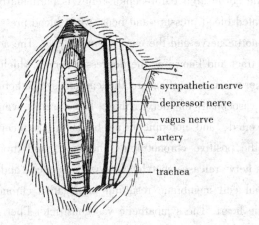

— sympathetic nerve
— depressor nerve
— vagus nerve
— artery
— trachea

Figure 5-9   Schematic diagram of cervical nerves and artery in rabbit

(4)Artery intubation: Tie the head end of the artery with a thread. Then clamp the body end of it with the artery clip. Cut a v-type hole near the head between the two ends with small scissors and insert the arterial cannula into the artery toward the heart. Tie the artery together with the cannula and fix the cannula by tying it around the branches. Remove the artery clip after you confirm that the artery is not bleeding.

(5)Connect the blood pressure transducer with the first channel of the signal acquisition system so as to record the blood pressure.

[**Observations**]

(1)Record the normal blood pressure curve. Identify the waves (Figure 5-10).

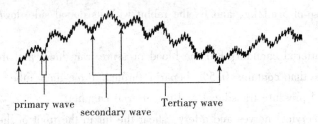

primary wave
secondary wave
Tertiary wave

Figure 5-10   The blood pressure curve of the common carotid artery in the rabbit

①Primary wave (heart beat wave): it is the fluctuation of blood pressure caused by ventricle systole and diastole. Cardiac contraction increases blood pressure and relaxation reduces it. Density of the wave denotes the heart rate. ②Secondary wave (respiration wave): it is the fluctuation of blood pressure caused by respiration movement. Blood pressure reduces and then increases during inspiration, but blood pressure increases and then reduces during expiration. ③Tertiary wave (seldom appears): the cause needs to be fully clarified, and it may be caused by the periodical changes of cardiovascular center tension.

(2) Clamp the other common carotid artery with the clip about 5-10 s. Then remove the clip. Record the changes of blood pressure and heart rate.

(3) Hold the thread which ligated the artery, pull the artery in the direction to the heart for 5-10 s. Record the changes of blood pressure and heart rate.

(4) Inject 1 ∶ 10 000 noradrenaline (NE) 0. 2-0. 3 ml, Record the changes of blood pressure and heart rate.

(5) Inject 1 ∶ 100 000 acetylcholine (ACh) 0. 2-0. 3 ml, Record the changes of blood pressure and heart rate.

(6) Inject atropine1 0. 5 ml, after 1-2 min inject 1 ∶ 100 000 acetylcholine (ACh) 0. 2-0. 3 ml, Record the changes of blood pressure and heart rate.

(7) Stimulate the depressor nerve with stimulating electrode (20 Hz and 3-5 V). Record the changes of blood pressure and heart rate. Ligate the depressor nerve with two threads. Cut the depressor nerve between the two ligations with small scissors. Stimulate the head end and body end of the nerve. Record the changes of blood pressure and heart rate.

(8) Ligate the right vagus nerve with two threads. Cut the nerve between the two ligations with small scissors. Stimulate the head end of the nerve with the stimulating electrode (20 Hz and 5-10 V) for 10 s. Record the changes of blood pressure and heart rate.

(9) Lift the head of the rabbit quickly and keep it up for 2-5 s. Record the changes of blood pressure and heart rate. Put the head down and lift the lower limbs of the rabbit quickly and keep it up for 2-5 s. Record the changes of blood pressure and heart rate.

[Notices]

(1) Proper anesthesia. Inadequate anesthesia will result in rabbit struggling; too deep anesthesia will result in insensitive reflection or even death of the rabbit.

(2) Artery cannula should be inserted at the same direction with the artery, so as to insure efficient transduction of blood pressure to the transducer and prevent blood vessel injury.

(3) After observation of each item, do next item until the blood pressure has resumed to normal.

(4) Protect the ear vein. Immediately inject 0. 5ml saline after drug injection to prevent drug remains in the needle and vein.

(5) Use a glass needle to separate nerves, do not pull the nerve too hard. Drip saline to keep the nerve wet.

[Question]

Discuss the mechanisms of the neural and humoral factors affecting blood pressure.

[Key Words]

heart rate   neural and humoral regulation

(Tong Zan)

Experiment 16   Discharge of Depressor Nerve in Rabbit

[**Purpose**]

(1) Learn the method of recording the discharge of nerves.

(2) Observe the characteristics of the discharge of depressor nerve in rabbit

[**Principle**]

The afferent nerve fiber of the aortic arch baroreceptor joins the vagus nerve reaching to medulla oblongata in most mammals. However, the afferent nerve fiber in rabbits remains an independent tract, in parallel with the vagus nerve and the sympathetic nerve. It is called depressor nerve. The depressor nerve plays an important role in regulation of arterial blood pressure. When the arterial blood pressure increases, baroreceptors transmit more signals into the central nervous system through the depressor nerve; and the blood pressure goes down. Conversely, when the arterial blood pressure decreases, baroreceptors transmit less signals into the central nerve system through depressor nerve; and the blood pressure goes up. Therefore, while the arterial blood pressure fluctuates in a cardiac cycle, the afferent impulse by depressor nerve shows periodical changes.

[**Objects**]

Rabbit.

[**Materials and Equipments**]

20% ethyl carbamate, heparin, 1 : 10 000 noradrenaline, 1 : 100 000 acetycholine, saline, liquid paraffin.

RM6240 physiological signal acquisition and processing system, operating instruments for mammal, loudspeaker box, blood pressure transducer, tracheal cannula, arterial cannula, artery clip, recording electrode, injectors, glass needle, gauze, fixing frames, thread.

[**Experimental Procedure**]

(1) Anesthesia and fixation of the animal: Inject 20% ethyl carbamate into the ear vein slowly with the dose of 5 ml/kg, and fix the rabbit with its dorsal side down on the operating table.

(2) Operation: Shear the fur in the front of the neck and cut the skin along the midline. Separate the trachea, and do tracheal intubation. Clamp the edge of the incision with hemostatic forceps; lift and turn outside the cervical tissue beside trachea using the index finger of the other hand; expose the vascular plexus. The depressor nerve is the thinnest nerve compared to the vagus and sympathetic nerve. Use a glass needle to separate the depressor nerve carefully and put a saline moistened thread under it.

(3) Artery intubation: Separate the common carotid artery, and do artery intubation (Method refers to Neural and Humoral Regulation of Circulatory System). Connect the blood

pressure transducer with the second channel of the signal acquisition system so as to record the blood pressure.

(4)Recording the discharge of the depressor nerve: Hook the depressor nerve using the recording electrode. Make the nerve impending, avoiding contact with the surrounding tissue. Fix the electrode on the frames. Make a bag with the surrounding skin, dripping some warm liquid paraffin on the nerve, so as to prevent the nerve from injury. Connect the recording electrode to the first channel of the signal acquisition system.

[**Observation Items**]

(1) Recording the discharge of the depressor nerve and blood pressure, observe the characteristic of the discharge of the depressor nerve(Figure 5-11).

(2) Connect signal acquisition system with loudspeaker box, you can hear the voice of the discharge of depressor nerve. It should be similar with the voice of the train.

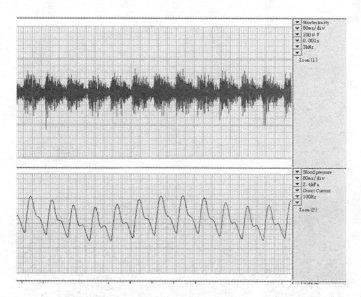

Figure 5-11   The discharge of depressor nerve and the arterial blood pressure

(3) Inject 1 : 100 000 acetylcholine (ACh) 0. 2-0. 3 ml, observe the frequency and range changes of the discharge and changes of blood pressure.

(4) After the blood pressure recovers to normal, inject 1 : 10 000 noradrenaline (NE) 0. 2-0. 3 ml, observe the frequency and range changes of the discharge and changes of blood pressure.

[**Attention**]

(1)Separate the nerves gently, and drip warm liquid paraffin in time once the nerves are separated. Avoid bleeding. If the voltage is reduced, move the recording electrode closer to the heart side.

(2)Avoid improper anesthesia. Avoid recording electrode contact with other tissues. Try to eliminate interference.

[**Question and Discussion**]

1. Describe the relationship between the discharge of the depressor nerve and the heartbeat or blood pressure.

2. Explain the mechanism of ACh and NE affecting the discharge of the depressor nerve.

[**Key Words**]

Depressor nerve   baroreceptor reflex

(Tong Zan)

Chapter 6   Respiration

Experiment 17   Vital Capacity Measurement

[Purpose]

To study measuring vital capacity by electronic spirometer

[Principle]

The main function of the lung is gas exchange to maintain normal metabolism. Vital capacity is the maximum amount of air a person can expel from the lungs after a maximum inhalation. It is equal to the sum of inspiratory reserve volume, tidal volume, and expiratory reserve volume. A person's vital capacity can be measured by a regular spirometer. In combination with other physiological measurements, the vital capacity can help make a diagnosis of underlying lung disease. A normal adult has a vital capacity between 3 and 5 liters. A human's vital capacity depends on age, gender, height, weight, and ethnicity.

[Objects]

Human beings.

[Materials and Equipments]

Electronic spirometer, disposable mouth piece.

[Experimental Procedures]

(1) The flow spirometer is used to measure exhalation of air. You must reset the dial to zero and use a fresh mouthpiece before each use. After you have used it then put it into the Milton solution.

(2) Take the deepest inspiration you can and exhale into it through a rubber tube to maximum capacity, letting all the air out. Read the volume on the screen of the Spirometer.

(3) Continues to test for a total of three times, recording the maximal volume as your vital capacity.

[Observations]

Record the volume readings from the spirometer and label the maximal one as your vital capacity.

vital capacity

	1st	2nd	3rd
vital capacity(ml)			

[Notices]

1. Avoid oxygen exchange through the nose

2. Use a disposable mouth piece.

[Questions]

Why is the maximal volume recorded as your vital capacity?

[Key Words]

vital capacity

(Peng Biwen)

Experiment 18   Discharge of Phrenic Nerve

[Purpose]

To study the method of recording the discharge of the phrenic nerve *in vivo*.

[Experimental Principle]

The basic rhythm of respiration is generated in the respiratory center. The respiratory center emits repetitive bursts of inspiratory action potential which is transmitted to primary respiratory muscles, mainly the diaphragm, through efferent nerves. So the discharge of the phrenic nerve that controls the diaphragm reflects the activity of the respiratory center. The nervous discharge is not an instantaneous burst of action potential. In normal respiration, it begins weakly and increases steadily in a ramp manner for about 2 seconds. It then ceases abruptly for approximately the next 3 seconds, which turns off the excitation of the diaphragm and allows elastic recoil of the lungs and the chest wall to cause expiration. Next, the inspiratory signal will begin again for another cycle; this cycle continues repeatedly, with expiration occurring in between cycles. In the experiment, the relationship between the discharge of the phrenic nerve and the phase of inspiration and expiration is observed by synchronous recording of the nervous discharge and the movement of the diaphragm.

[Objects]

Rabbit.

[Materials and Equipments]

(1)Solutions: 20% ethyl carbamate, liquid paraffin.

(2)Equipment: protective electrode, operating instruments of mammalian, iron stand, biconcave clamp, operating table of rabbit, tracheal cannula, rubber tube, syringe (10,

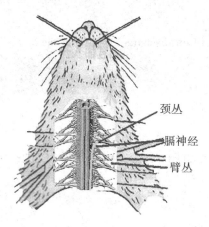

颈丛

膈神经

臂丛

Figure 6-1

20ml), surgical needle, colored silk thread(Figure 6-1).

[**Procedures**]

1. Anesthesia and Fixation

Weigh rabbit: 20% ethyl carbamate (1g/kg) is injected into the vein in the edge of the ear. After the disappearance of the corneal reflex, fix the rabbit on the operating table, and turn on the light at the table bottom to keep constant temperature.

2. Operation

Shear the hair on the neck, cut the skin along the middle cervical line and separate the trachea with hemostats. Cut down the trachea, insert the tracheal cannula, and then fix the trachea with thread. Separate both sides of the vagus nerve, securing two threads under them. Pull apart the skin and muscles above the trachea with hemostats, locating the brachial nerve which is rooted vertical to the vertebral column. The phrenic nerve goes along the spine and crosses the root of the brachial nerve. Separate the phrenic nerve for 1-2 cm and put a silk thread under it. Fill the 38℃ liquid paraffin into the interspaces around the phrenic nerve to protect the nerve.

[**Observations**]

(1) Record the normal discharge of the phrenic nerve and the curves of respiratory movement. Distinguish the phase of inspiration and expiration, observing the nerve discharge. Monitor the sound of nerve discharge.

(2) The effect of vagus nerve on discharge of phrenic nerve: cut off one side of the vagus nerve, observing the changes of discharge in the phrenic nerve. Then cut off the other vagus nerve and observe the changes of discharge in the phrenic nerve.

[**Notices**]

(1) Carefully separate nerves to prevent injuring them.

(2) Fill the 38℃ liquid paraffin into the interspaces around the phrenic nerve to protect

the nerve.

[**Questions**]

What effect of vagus nerve on discharge of phrenic nerve?

[**Key Words**]

phrenic nerve

(Peng Biwen)

Experiment 19   Pleural Negative Pressure and Pneumothorax

[**Purpose**]

To verify the existence of intrapleural pressure; To learn how to measure it; To learn how to make artificial pneumothorax.

[**Principle**]

In physiology, intrapleural pressure (also called intrathoracic pressure) refers to the pressure within the pleural cavity. Normally, the pressure within the pleural cavity is slightly less than the atmospheric pressure, in what is known as negative pressure. When the pleural cavity is damaged/ruptured and the intrapleural pressure becomes equal to or exceeds the atmospheric pressure, pneumothorax may ensue.

[**Objects**]

Rabbit.

[**Materials and Equipments**]

surgical instruments; operating table; pneumothorax needle, U shape water column manometer, trachea cannula.

[**Procedures**]

(1) Anesthesia: Weigh the rabbit. The rabbit is anesthetized by 20% urethane injection (5ml/kg) in an ear vein.

(2) Animal fixation: Secure the legs and arms of the rabbit in a knot and fix to the operating table. Place a butterfly type loop around each limb and tie them so tightly that the animals' body is motionless.

(3) Operation: Shear the hair on the neck. Open the skin with a scalpel, making a mid-incision 4-6 cm with the scalpel over the region from the lower jaw to the breastbone. Separate the muscles in the front of the thorax, then separate the trachea.

(4) Tracheal intubation: Pass a thread under the trachea, making a "T" shape incision on it under the throat, then insert the tracheal cannula toward the lung and tie the cannula and the trachea together.

(5) Connect the respiratory transducer to a computerized acquisition and management instrument for biological signals.

(6) The right lungs of the anesthetized rabbits were penetrated with a sterilized 19G needle on the lower edge of the 4th rib.

[**Observations**]

To observe the fluctuation on the surface of water column manometer, plug the needle liganding with the water-pressure instrument into the pleural cavity, observing the change of layer of the fluid during the course of respiratory movement.

[**Notices**]

Carefully separate tissue to prevent injuring.

[**Thinking and Evaluation**]

Why is the intrapleural pressure negative compared to the barometric pressure?

[**Key Words**]

intrapleural pressure   pneumothorax

(Peng Biwen)

Experiment 20   Respiratory Regulation

[**Experimental Consideration and Aim**]

To study the method of respiratory movement recordings in the rabbit; Observe and analyze the influence of pulmonary stretch reflex or other factors on respiratory movement.

[**Experimental Principle**]

Due to the regulatory mechanism in our body, respiratory movement of human and other mammals can be persistent, and rhythmically proceed. Different kinds of stimuli *in vivo* or *in vitro* can directly effect the main center or different parts of the sensors and influence respiratory movement for the needs of the metabolism of the body. Pulmonary stretch reflex participates in the regulation of breathing rhythm.

[**Objects**]

Rabbit.

[**Medicine and Equipment**]

Operating table; surgical instruments; tension sensor; 20ml and 5ml injection syringe; rubber tube (length 50cm inner diameter 1cm); 20% ethyl urethane; saline; 3% lactic acid; CO_2 air bag; soda lime air bag.

[**Procedures**]

1. Exclusion of Xiphoid cartilage

Cut off the xiphoid skin of the sternum extremitas inferior, then make an incision about 2 cm long along the linea alba. Separating the tissue on the face of xiphoid carefully (don't injury the chest), expose the xiphoid cartilage and bone hilt, cutting out a length of bone hilt with crown scissors to separate the xiphoid and sternum completely. You must reserve the diaphragm piece under it and keep it intact. Then the movement of diaphragm will affect the xiphoid cartilage.

2. Secure a metal hook tied with a long string to the center part of the free xiphoid cartilage, with the other end of the string related to the strain beam of the tension sensor through the universal pulley.

3. Start the computer acquisition system and connect to the tension sensor input channel adjusting the recording system to make the breathing curve clearly displayed on the screen.

[**Observations**]

(1) Record the respiratory movement curve, identify carefully the relationship of curve and breath in or out.

(2) The influence of CO_2 on breathing.

Connect a bypath of the trachea intubation tube to an air bag filled with CO_2 and clamp the other bypath to ensure the rabbit is breathing from the bag. Observe and record the change of respiratory movement. If a significant change appears, loosen the hemostatic forceps immediately and remove the rubber tube to get the breathing right.

(3) The influence of hypoxia on breathing.

Connect a bypath of the trachea intubation tube to an air bag filled with soda lime, and clamp the other bypath. Observe and record the change of the respiratory movement curve. If a significant change appears, loosen the hemostatic forceps immediately and remove the rubber tube to get the breathing right.

(4) The effect of increase the dead space on breathing.

Connect a rubber tube to a bypath of the trachea intubation tube, then use a hemostatic forcep to clamp the other bypath to increase the dead space. Observe and record the change of the respiratory movement curve. Once a significant change appears, loosen the hemostatic forceps immediately and remove the rubber tube to get the breathing right.

(5) The effect of increase the airway resistance on the breathing.

After breathing has returned to normal, clamp the two bypaths for several seconds and observe respiratory changes.

(6) The influence of lactic acid on breathing.

Inject 1ml 3% lactic acid from ear vein, then observe and record the change of respiratory movement.

(7) Pulmonary stretch reflex.

After being returned to normal breathing, connect a bypath of the trachea intubation tube to a 20ml syringe, and inject 20ml of air. When the breathing gets smooth, slowly inject 20ml of air into the lung with three times that of the normal breathing rhythm and clamp the other bypath. Observe the change of respiratory rhythm and breathing state. Release the bypath immediately after the experiment and breathing begins to normalize. In the same way, extract air from the lung at the end of the expiration; observe the difference between expiration and inspiration. (Note: if the injection and extraction is limited to three times of breathing rate, then release the bypath immediately)

(8) After being returned to normal breathing, ligature bilateral vagus (operate at the same time and ligature tightly, ensuring to block the transmission of nerve impulses). Observe and record the change of respiratory movement before and after ligation. Cut down the bilateral vagus nerves, stimulating the central end and the peripheral end. Observe and record the change of the respiratory movement curve.

[Tips]

(1) Each item needs its control.

(2) Set proper stimulation intensity on the vagus nerve .

[Questions]

According to the experimental item7 observation, why is demand of gas injection and extraction time limited to three normal breathing rhythms?

[Key Words]

pulmonary stretch reflex

(Wan Shuxia)

Chapter 7   Gastrointestinal Physiology

Experiment 21   Movement of Intestine Muscle in Vitro

[Purpose]

The purpose of this experiment is to master the experimental methods of the organs of warm-blooded animals in vitro. Also, observe general characteristics of gastrointestinal smooth muscle in rabbit and the effect of adrenalin, Ach, HCl, NaOH and $CaCl_2$ on rabbit's intestine *in vitro*.

[Principle]

The smooth muscle in the digestive tract has its own specific characteristics, such as lower excitability, slow contraction, extension, tension, auto-rhythmicity, sensitivity to stimulators of chemistry, temperature and mechanical stretch, and not only have the excitability, conductivity, and contractility as same as skeletal muscle and myocardium. These characteristics of the smooth muscle in the digestive tract are important to maintain pressure in the digestive tract, keep certain form and position of gastrointestinal tract, and suit to physical and chemical change of substances in the digestive tract. The action of the smooth muscle in the digestive tract is adjusted by the central nervous system and humoral factors *in vivo*. In order to observe characteristics of smooth muscle in the digestive tract of mammals, intestine muscle in vitro must be put in suitable environment that is near to *in vivo* conditions. Tyrodo's solution is selected as an infusing solution in the experiment because its composition is similar to that of the rabbit's body liquid. Keep infusing solution temperature at about 37℃ and input oxygen to Tyrodo's solution constantly during the experiment.

[Object]

Rabbit.

[Materials and Equipments]

1. Solutions: Tyrodo's solution, 0.9% NaCl, 1 : 10 000 adrenaline, 1 : 10 000 ACh, 1 : 10 000(g/ml) atropine, 1 mol/L NaOH, 1mol/L HCl, 1% $CaCl_2$.

2. Equipment: tension transducer, super homoeothermic water bath, operating instruments for toad, dropper, mortar and pounder, oxygen generator or oxygen balloon, coiled condenser and condenser clamps, iron support, beaker, glass stick , bath dish, bath tube, syringe (1

ml), test tube and holder, rubber tube, cotton thread.

[Experimental Procedures]

1. Emplace super homoeothermic water bath device

Use tap water to fill the bath of the thermostatic bath device, and Tyrodo's solution into the pre-liquid pipe and specimen slot, and then set the temperature of super homoeothermic water bath at 37 ±0.5℃. Adjust air input of specimen slot. [Figure 6-2]

2. Preparation of a rabbit's intestine sample in vitro

(1) The rabbit was knocked dizzy by a blow on the head. Pieces of rabbit duodenum (10-15 cm from the pylorus) were removed, freed from mesenteric attachment and washed with Precooling of Tyrodo's solution (4℃), and cut into smaller segments (2-3 cm).

(2) Ligate respectively at both opposite angles of the length of intestine wall with thread and needle after cleaning. Superior thread is connected with the strain patch of a tension transducer, and inferior thread is fixed in bottom of the specimen slot. Segments were allowed to equilibrate in Tyrode solution for 20 min before recording experiment.

3. Connection of equipment: Connect the signal input lead of intension transducer to channel 1 of RM6240 or BL-420E systems, and then enter the experimental operating system. Adjust recording speed, baseline, and relative parameters.

[Observations]

1. Observe the rhythmic movement of the intestine smooth muscle in normal Tyrodo's solution.

2. Add adrenaline (1 : 10000) 1-2 drops to specimen slot. Observe and record the changes of tension and contraction of the intestine. Discharge the solution fluid in the specimen slot and clean it three times with Tyrodo's solution after an obvious change of the rhythmic movement of intestine muscle was observed.

3. Add ACh (1 : 10000) 1-2 drops to the specimen slot and observe the changes of intestine activity. Discharge the solution fluid in specimen slot and clean it three times with Tyrodo's solution after an obvious change of intestine activity was observed.

4. Add atropine (1 : 10000) 2-4 drops to the specimen slot, after 2min, add ACh (1 : 10000) 1-2 drops to the specimen slot and observe the changes of intestine activity. Compare this result with the result of the above third. Clean specimen slot as above.

5. Add 1% $CaCl_2$ 1-2 drops to specimen slot. Observe the changes of intestine activity. Clean specimen slot as above.

6. Add 1ml/L HCl 1-2 drops to specimen slot. Observe the effect on the intestine. Then add 1ml/L NaOH 1-2 drops to specimen slot. Observe the changes of intestine activity. Clean specimen slot as above.

7. Exchange solution in specimen slot with 25℃ Tyrodo's solution and observe the changes of intestine activity, gradually warming up to 38 ℃ to further observe the changes of intestine activity.

[**Notices**]

(1) Prepare 37℃ Tyrodo's solution for exchange before adding drugs.

(2) Exchange solution in bath tube and clean it three times with Tyrodo's solution after the effect of drug was observed. After the activity of intestine muscle has recovered, please observe next item.

(3) Tyrodo's solution in specimen slot must be higher than the intestine sample and be controlled at the same height during the experiment.

(4) O_2 must be added during the whole experiment and be controlled at 2-3 air bubbles per second. Excessive bubbling may affect recording result.

(5) Prevent each drug from being added excessively at one time to cause irreversible reaction.

(6) The reagent dropper must to be dedicated to avoid contamination.

[**Question**]

1. Why is the upper segment of the small intestine taken, especially the duodenal muscle segment, in preparing small intestine smooth muscle specimens?

2. What conditions are required for in vitro experimentation for tissues and organs of mammals?

3. What are the main physiological characteristics of smooth muscles in the digestive tract in this experiment? Explain the phenomena observed in the experiment.

4. What difference is there in the effect of adrenaline and acetylcholine on the small intestine smooth muscle and cardiac muscle?

5. Why not use of rabbit small intestine after anesthesia, but rather use of the stun rabbit small intestine in the experiment?

[**Key Words**]

gastrointestinal smooth muscle	excitability
contractility	autorhythmicity
extensibility	tonicity

(Yan Xiaohong)

Experiment 22　Observation of Gastrointestinal Motility in Vivo

[**Purpose**]

The aim of this experiment is to observe the gastrointestinal motility and learn the regulation effect of neural and humoral factors on the movement of the gastrointestinal tract.

[**principle**]

In the process of food digestion, contraction of smooth muscles in the gastrointestinal tract wall serves to mix the luminal contents with the various secretions, and move the contents through the tract from mouth to anus. These contractions are referred to the motility of the gastrointestinal tract. Functional types of movements in the gastrointestinal tract include mainly tonic contraction, peristalsis, the gastric receptive relaxation, and the intestinal segmentation contraction. The motility of the gastrointestinal tract is under neural control both by the autonomic nervous system and the enteric nervous system.

The gastrointestinal tract has its own local nervous system, known as the enteric nervous system. The cell bodies and their nerve fibers, and nerve fibers from extrinsic nerves constitute the enteric nervous system. The enteric nervous system contains adrenergic and cholinergic neurons as well as neurons that release other neurotransmitters.

The autonomic nervous system, also termed extrinsic nervous system, includes the sympathetic nerve and parasympathetic nerve. The fibers of sympathetic nerves, whose postganglionic actions are mediated by norepinephrine (NE), reach the gut via the splanchnic nerves and inhibit gastrointestinal tract motility. Parasympathetic nerves includes the vagus nerve and pelvic nerve. The action of postganglionic fibers of parasympathetic nerves to smooth muscle is mainly mediated by the muscarinic action of acetylcholine (Ach), which is blocked by the atropine and stimulates gastrointestinal tract motility. Acetylcholine most often excites gastrointestinal activity, and the norepinephrine, almost always inhibits gastrointestinal activity.

[**Object**]

Rabbit.

[**Materials and Equipments**]

(1) **Equipments**: protective electrode, operating instruments of mammal, operating table of rabbit, glass dissociative needle, gauze, Syringe (20ml and 1ml).

(2) **Solution**: 20% Ethyl Carbamate (Urethan), Tyrode's solution(or 0.9%NaCl), 1 : 10 000 epinephrine, neostigmine (1mg/ml), 1 : 10 000 Ach, atropine (0.5mg/ml).

[**Methods**]

1. Anesthesia

Fixation and skin preparation of rabbit: Capture the rabbit, weigh it and calculate the dose of anesthesia; inject 20% Ethyl Carbamate (5ml/kg) into the rabbit's marginal ear vein. Fix the anesthetized rabbit on the operation table and let it lie on its back. Shear the hair on the neck and abdomen.

2. Operation

(1) Intubate the trachea: Cut the fur and make a 4-5 cm neck incision; separate the muscles by blunt dissection; expose the trachea and put a thread under it; cut the trachea, using a "T" incision under thyroid cartilage and insert a tracheal cannula into it and ligate it.

(2) Cut the abdomen 8-10 cm using a median incision at about 0.5 cm below the xiphoid, and expose the stomach and intestines.

(3) Find the anterior branches of the subdiaphragmatic vagus nerve at the end of the esophagus and the greater splanchnic nerve at the upper end of adrenal gland in left lateral

abdominal posterior wall. Pass a thread respectively for further experiment.

3. Connection of equipment

Connect protective electrode and the output lead of stimulus from RM6240 system, and then enter experimental operating system.

[**Observation items**]

(1) Observe the movement patterns of the gastrointestinal tract, pay attention to the peristalsis, tonic contraction, and segmental contraction.

(2) Stimulate the subdiaphragmatic vagus nerve (0. 2ms, 2-5V, 20-30Hz) for 1-3 min, observing the changes of the gastrointestinal motility.

(3) Inject the atropine 0.5 mg into the marginal ear vein, then stimulate the subdiaphragmatic vagus nerve (0. 2ms, 2-5V, 20-30Hz) for 1-3 min, observing the changes of the gastrointestinal motility.

(4) Inject the neostigmine 0. 1-0. 2 mg into the marginal ear vein, observing the changes of the gastrointestinal motility.

(5) Inject the epinephrine (1 : 10 000) 0. 5 ml into the marginal ear vein, observing the changes of the gastrointestinal motility.

(6) Inject the ACh (1 : 10 000) 0. 5 ml into the marginal ear vein, observing the changes of the gastrointestinal motility.

(7) Stimulate the greater splanchnic nerve (0. 2ms, 2-5V, 20-30Hz) for 1-3 min, observing the changes of the gastrointestinal motility.

[**Notices**]

(1) Please keep the gastrointestinal moist using the tepid Tyrode's solution during the experiment. If the gastrointestinal tract was exposed to air too long, the movement of it will be weakened because of the dryness in the surface or the decrease of temperature of the tract.

(2) After one experimental item is performed, the effect was seen in a few minutes. After the gastrointestinal movements recover, please observe next item.

(3) Don't draw stomach and intestine excessively in process of operating .

[**Question**]

1. What are the patterns of gastrointestinal motility in the rabbit? How to observe them?

2. How to disassociate the subdiaphragmatic vagus nerve and the greater splanchnic nerve?

3. When the vagus and the greater splanchnic nerve are stimulated, are the gastrointestinal motility effects shown to be converse with the expected results? Why?

[**Key Words**]

gastrointestinal motility	tonic contraction
receptive relaxation	peristalsis
segmentation contraction	parasympathetic nerve
sympathetic nerve	acetylcholin, Ach
noradrenalin, NA	

(Yan Xiaohong)

Experiment 23   Regulation of Bile Secretion in Rabbits

[**Purposes**]

　　(1) To study and master the method of common bile duct intubation and bile drainage

　　(2) To observe the effects of neuro-humoral factors on bile secretion.

[**Principles**]

　　Bile is excreted by hepatocytes continuously and is drained out through hepatic ducts. Owing to the contraction of Oddi's sphincter in the interdigestive stage, bile is prevented from excreting into the duodenum and is stored up in the gallbladder. In the digestive stage, the bile excreted directly by hepatocytes and stored in gallbladder is drained into the duodenum due to the relaxation of Oddi's sphincter and promotes the digestion and absorption of fatty substances. Many factors are involved in bile excretion. Food is a natural stimulus for hepatocytes to excrete bile. The exciting of the vagus nerves and many humoral factors such as gastrin, secretin, cholecystokinin and bile salt all regulate bile excretion via promoting hepatocytes activity and/or facilitating the contraction of the gallbladder and the relaxation of Oddi's sphincter. In addition, the declined pH value in the small intestine can foster bile excretion via increasing the release of the secretin.

[**Object**]

　　Rabbit (body weight 2-2.5 kg).

[**Materials and Equipments**]

　　(1) Solutions: saline, 20% ethyl carbamate, 1 : 100 000 Ach, 0.1mol/L HCl.

　　(2) Equipment: operating table for rabbit, operating instruments, electrostimulation apparatus, syringe (10ml, 5ml and 1 ml), fine plastic tube, beaker, protective electrode, RM-6240 biological signal recording system.

[**Methods**]

　　1. Anesthesia

　　The rabbit is anesthetized with 20% ethyl carbamate or 3% sodium pentobarbital before surgery. The injection volume is lg/kg for intravenous route by marginal auricular vein. After anesthesia, the rabbit is fixed on the rabbit operation table on its back.

　　2. Operation on Neck

　　The rabbit is sheared on the neck, and the skin of the neck is cut along the midline. Subcutaneous tissues and muscle tissues are separated to expose the trachea. Cut the trachea and intubate the tracheal cannula.

　　3. Operation on Abdomen and Intubation of Common Bile Duct

　　①The rabbit is sheared on the upper abdomen. ②The skin of the upper abdomen is cut along the midline below the xiphoid, and the incision is about 7-10cm long. The abdominal cavity is opened. ③The anterior branch of the vagus under diaphragm is separated and a silk thread is put beneath the nerve branch. ④ About 1ml of bile is taken out of the gallbladder. ⑤ The duodenum can be found at the end of pylorus, and the common bile duct, a major muscular duct that appears yellow and green can be found on the back of the superior extremity of duodenum. ⑥The common bile duct next to the duodenum is dissociated and a piece of thread is put beneath it. ⑦A minor incision is made on the common bile duct next to the duodenum and a fine plastic tube is inserted into the duct and fixed by ligaturing. ⑧ Cover the surgical wound with warm wet gauze.

4. Collection of Bile

The bile is collected with a beaker.

5. Connections of Apparatus

Connect the input cable with the channel 1 of the biological signal recording apparatus. Adjust recording electrodes and make sure that the bile drops out of cannula and touchs the recording electrodes while falling down.

[**Observation Items**]

(1) Observe the normal bile secretion, and count the drops of bile per minute.

(2) Stimulating the vagus nerve discontinuously with medium intensity (5-10V) and frequency (20-30Hz) for 1 minute, repeat twice with 2 minutes interval, and then observe the latent period and the volume of bile secretion.

(3) Inject 1ml of 1 : 10 000 Ach into marginal ear vein and observe the latent period and the volume of bile secretion.

(4) Dilute the gallbladder bile with saline according to 1 : 10. Inject 5ml dilute bile into marginal ear vein and observe the latent period and the volume of bile secretion.

(5) Ligating two ends of duodenum and fill 20 ml of 37℃ 0.1mol/L HCl in it, and then observe the latent period and the volume of bile secretion.

[**Notices**]

(1) The injury of associated blood vessels and nerves should be avoided when dissociating common bile duct. If bleeding, please take some hemostatic measures in time.

(2) The incision of the common bile duct should be close to the duodenum.

(3) The inserted tube should be kept parallel to the common bile duct to prevent the duct from piercing.

(4) The incision of the abdomen is covered with warm gauze dipped in saline during recording.

[**Questions**]

1. How to explain the phenomenon that the bile flows out fast soon after the intubation of the common bile duct, then the flowing speed slows down and inclines to be stable.

2. What is the mechanism of bile secretion by stimulating the vagus?

3. Which ingredient in the bile can influence bile secretion? And how does it affect bile

secretion under the normal physiological conditions?

[**Key Words**]

    bile seeretion

(Chen Taoxiang)

Chapter 8　Kidney

Experiment 24　Factors Influencing the Urine Formation in Rabbits

[**Purposes**]

(1) To learn the usage of ureter cannula or bladder cannula, and master the method of collecting urine

(2) To observe influencing factors on urine volume and some components in urine, and then analyze their mechanisms

[**Principles**]

The procedure of urine formation includes the filtration in renal glomcrulus, the reabsorption and excretion in renal tubules and collecting duct. Any factor that affects the procedure of urine formation could alter urine volume and /or the components of urine.

[**Object**]

Rabbits with body weight 2-2. 5 kg.

[**Materials and Equipments**]

(1) Drugs: 20% ethyl carbamate or 3% sodium pentobarbital, 50% glucose, 0. 9% sodium chloride, 1 : 10 000 noradrcnaline, pituitrin, furosemide, 0. 6% phenol red, 10% sodium hydroxide, heparin, indicator paper of urine sugar;

(2) Instruments: RM6240 biological signal recording system, pressure transducer, mammalian surgical instruments, bladder cannula or ureter cannula, artery cannula, fine plastic cannula, instrument of collecting urine, artery clip, stimulating electrodes, syringes (20ml, 10ml, 5ml, 1ml), syringe needles, tubes, tubes stand, alcoholic burner, culture disks, operating-lamp, gauze, cotton ropes, silk thread, operating table.

[**Methods**]

1. Surgery on Animals

(1) Anesthesia and fixation: I. V. 20% ethyl carbamate (1g/kg) or 3% sodium pentobarbital (30-40mg/kg) into the vein of the marginal ear to anesthetize the rabbit, and fix it on the operating table in supine position.

(2)Tracheal intubation and arterial intubation: Shear the hair covering the neck to expose operating field, perform surgical operation on the neck to intubate tracheal cannula. Separate the left common artery and the right vagus nerve respectively. Arterial intubation: place two silk threads beneath the common artery, fasten the distal end of the common artery with one silk thread, and clamp the proximal end with artery clip. Make a bevel incision on the common artery close to the knot, intubate the arterial cannula filled with heparinized saline, fasten and fix the cannula with the other silk thread, and loosen the artery clip.

(3) Urine collection: the methods of collecting urine are as follows: Shear the hair on the inferior belly, make an upward incision 5cm long on the abdominal skin along the midline from the upper edge of the pubic symphysis, and open the abdominal wall and peritoneum with surgical scissors along the linea alba. Drag the bladder out of the abdominal cavity, put the apex of bladder upward and expose the trigone of the bladder. Locate the bilateral ureters and discern their entrances to the bladder.

①Bladder intubation: Place a silk thread beneath the bilateral ureters, turn the bladder upward, and ligate the urethra. Circle the bladder wall with a few vessels with purse string suture, and keep two terminals of suture. Make a small incision on the bladder wall just within the center of the circle, intubate the bladder cannula, and fasten and fix it with two terminals of suture. After the operation, cover the wound with the gauze soaked with warm saline buffer. Make sure that the urine just drops to the recording electrodes by adjusting the orientation of the bladder cannula.

②Ureter intubation: Separate the ureters from neighboring tissues and place two silk threads beneath each ureter. Ligate the left ureter near the bladder with one silk thread to block urine's influx. Make a small V-shape incision on the ureter just above the knot, intubate the ureter cannula filled with saline buffer, and fasten and fix it with the other silk thread. Do the same operations to the right ureter. After the operation, cover the wound with the gauze soaked with warm saline buffer. Make sure that the urine just drops on the recording electrodes by adjusting the orientation of the ureter cannula.

2. Setup of the instruments

Connect the channel 1 with the guide line for drop signal and connect channel 2 with the guide line of the pressure transducer.

[**Experimental Items**]

(1) Record the relatively normal blood pressure curve and urine volume in a condition without any treatment.

(2) I. V. 37℃ 0.9% sodium chloride 30 ml quickly (within a minute), and observe the changes of blood pressure and urine volume.

(3) I. V. 1 : 10 000 noradrenaline 0.3-0.5 ml, and observe the changes of blood pressure and urine volume.

(4) Take two drops of urine and test the glucose level by indicator paper of urine sugar. Then I. V. 50% glucose solution 2 ml, and observe the changes of blood pressure and urine volume. After urine volume has increased apparently, take two drops of urine and test the

glucose level again.

（5）I. V. pituitrin 2U, and observe the changes of blood pressure and urine volume.

（6）I. V. furosemide 0.5ml/kg, and observe the changes of blood pressure and urine volume.

（7）I. V. 0.6% phenol red solution 0.5ml and record the time "1". Collect urine with the culture disk containing 10% sodium hydroxide. Once phenol red is excreted by the kidneys and binds with sodium hydroxide, the solution shows purple red, record the time "2". Calculate the interval between time "1" and time "2", which means the interval from the time point of phenol red entering blood to the time point of its excretion out of the body. If ureter cannula or bladder cannula is too long, the time spending on phenol red's passing the cannula could not be ignored.

（8）Stimulation of the vagus nerve: ligate the right vagus nerve, cut it, and then stimulate its distal end with electric pulses discontinuously (stimulus intensity: 5-10V, frequency: 20-50Hz) for a minute. 3 seconds break follows 5 seconds-stimulation. Observe the changes of blood pressure and urine volume.

（9）Separate one femoral artery, make an incision on it and intubate a fine plastic cannula into the artery, letting blood out to maintain blood pressure in about 50 mmHg or so. Observe the changes of blood pressure and urine volume. Then I. V. 0.9% sodium chloride and observe the changes of blood pressure and urine volume.

[Notices]

（1）Feed the rabbit vegetables multiple times before the experiment in order to ensure that the rabbit is able to excrete enough urine during the experiment.

（2）Pay attention to protect the rabbit's vein on the edge of ear to ensure a good pathway for the injections.

（3）Perform experimental items step by step: The next item could not begin until the effects of the current item has disappeared.

（4）Experimental items are arranged according to the following rules: perform the item decreasing urine volume on basis of enough urine, and perform the item increasing urine volume on basis of little urine.

（5）Collect urine with a new container after injecting 50% glucose solution for test of urine sugar (if not, drip urine to indicator paper of urine sugar directly).

（6）In the item of stimulating the vagus nerve, select adequate stimulus intensity; don't stimulate the nerve with strong current continuously.

（7）Keep the animal warm in cold weather.

[Questions]

1. Among the influencing factors of urine formation in this experiment, which affect filtration in the renal glomerulus? Which affect reabsorption and excretion in renal tubules and the collecting duct?

2. What is the mechanism of the effect of stimulating the vagus nerve on urine volume?

[**Key Words**]

urine formation

(Chen Taoxiang)

Chapter 9　Sensory Physiology

Experiment 25　Visual Acuity

[Purpose]

(1) To learn how to test the visual acuity using standard logarithm vision chart.

(2) To test color vision by chart.

[Principle]

Visual acuity is the ability of the eye to distinguish the smallest details in space. A visual acuity threshold below which an object will go undetected. That is to say, there is a limitation of the visual acuity, expressed using the smallest image in the retina. The smallest image in the retina which can be distinguished by a normal eye is approximately as small as the average diameter of cones (1.5 μm) in the fovea of the retina.

The observer's task is to determine the orientation of the target (E or ℃). In all cases, the distinguishing feature is 1 unit in size. The size of the unit is varied to give a range of letter sizes, and the angular subtense of the unit at the eye is the minimum angle of resolution. The standard definition of normal visual acuity is the ability to resolve a spatial pattern separated by a visual angle of 1 minute of arc.

Color-blindness is the inability to distinguish the differences between certain colors.

[Objects]

Human beings.

[Materials and Equipments]

Logarithm vision chart.

[Experimental Procedures]

(1) Observers and subjects experimental in a light room.

(2) Put down your glasses and cover the eye of one side.

(3) Stand at a distance about 6 meters from the chart.

(4) Read the eye chart line of letters from large to small. At the left of each line you will find the approximate visual acuity, expressed in logarithm, which would be necessary to read the letters.

(5) Repeat for the other eye.

[**Notices**]

Keep enough light to read by.

[**Questions**]

1. Why is there a limitation of the visual acuity for our eyes?

2. What is color-blindness and its reason?

[**Key Words**]

Visual acuity color blindness

(Peng Biwen)

Experiment 26   Visual Accommodation and Pupillary Light Reflex

[**Purpose**]

Observe the visual accommodation and pupillary light reflex.

[**Principle**]

Looking at a target from far to near, or from near to far, human eye will experience an accommodation reflex. When looking the target from far to near, the convexity of crystalline lense increases, miosis and binocular convergence take place; otherwise it is the opposite change. The human eye miosis by light stimulation is called the pupillary light reflex. The experimental application of a spherical mirror imaging law to prove that near vision eye refraction system regulation is mainly the increase of the anterior lens surface convexity, while observing the miosis phenomenon with near objects and light stimuli.

[**Objects**]

Human beings.

[**Materials and Equipments**]

Candles, matches, flashlight.

[**Experimental Procedures**]

Observers and subjects do the experiment in a dark room.

[**Observations**]

(1) Place a lighted candle in the eye before subjects, and the subjects watch from several meters outside the goal. Experimenter can observe the three candle image in the subject (Figure 9-2). One of the brightest, medium-sized erect image is made by the front surface reflection of the cornea. The pupil can be seen in a dark and large erect image, the result of the reflection from the front surface of the lens. Another lighter and the smallest inverted image is the reflection of the lens rear surface is formed. The front surface of the cornea and lens are convex forward, therefore the erect image is formed; lens front surface curvature is smaller than the curvature of the anterior corneal surface, so the image is larger and darker. The posterior surface is concave forward, and its image is inverted, small, and light.

(2) The subjects gaze at 15cm of the candle, the largest figure seen at this time as to erect image brightest near and smaller. This shows that when near vision convex front surface of the lens increases closer to the cornea, the curvature becomes large, while the anterior corneal surface and the posterior surface curvature and position were not significantly changed. This is the adjustment of the eye reflex.

(3) Looking at near objects in a subject, you can still see miosis, eyes converging toward the nasal side, the former said pupil reflex, the latter said convergence reflex.

(4) The subject watches from afar, to observe the pupil size. Subjects were irradiated with a flashlight, visible light eye pupil shrink immediately. In order to prevent light irradiation the nasal blocking the other eye, repeat the test, while visible eyes pupillary shrink at the same time, called consensual light reflex.

[Notices]

(1) This test shall be carried out in a dark room

(2) After the flashlight illuminates the subject's eye, check the pupillary light reflex. Subjects should rest for 5 min to repeat, in order to prevent eye fatigue.

[Questions]

What is a candle imaging in the subjects eyes, respectively?

[Key Words]

Pupillary light reflex   convergence reflex

(Peng Biwen)

Experiment 27   Mapping the Blind Spot

[Purpose]

To test the blind spot in the vision field. Blind spot is an area on the retina without receptors to respond to light.

[Principle]

The blind spot is an area on the retina where the optic nerve and blood vessels enter and leave the retina, and hence where there are no rods or cones for visual reception, and a small object in the field of vision's blind spot becomes invisible. So, the human eye has a blind spot in its field of vision.

According to the principle of direct proportion between the corresponding line of two analogical triangles, we can calculate the diameter of a blind spot on the retina using the following formula: Diameter of blind spot on retina (Dr), Diameter of blind spot in the visual field (Dvf)

$$Dr = Dvf \times \frac{\text{distance from node to retina (15cm)}}{\text{distance from node to the paper (50cm)}}$$

[**Objects**]

Human beings.

[**Materials and equipments**]

Pencil, paper

[**Experimental procedures**]

A piece of paper is stuck on the wall.

[**Observations**]

(1) Testee keeps the right eye about 50 cm from the paper. Close the left eye and keep the head horizontal. Focus the right eye on the cross (Figure 9-3).

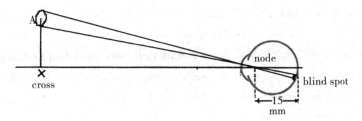

Figure 9-3

(2) Tester move a pencil slowly outward until it disappears in the visual field of the testee. When the tip disappears, tester will place a dot on the paper. Slowly move the tip of pencil until it appears in the visual field of the testee again, and place a dot on the paper.

(3) Connect the two dots, and then move the pencil from midpoint at a different angle, again placing a dot on the paper (generally make 8 dots), until a map of the area where testee cannot see is made. This area is the blind spot of the right eye of the testee.

(4) Repeat for the other eye

[**Notices**]

Keep the test eye staring at the cross, do not move the eye along with the tip of pencil in motion.

[**Questions**]

Is there a blind spot in our normal visual field for each eye? Why?

[**Key Words**]

visual field   visual acuity   blind spot

(Peng Biwen)

Experiment 28   Pathways of Sound Conduction

[**Purpose**]

(1) To learn how to use a tuning fork to generate sound.

(2) To understand the function of the auditory organ.

(3) To understand the pathways of sound conduction.

[**Principle**]

(1) **Hearing loss** occurs when there is loss of sound sensitivity produced by an abnormality in the auditory system. A wide variety of conditions can cause hearing loss. While physicians can sometimes identify its causes, in some cases the causes are unknown.

(2) **Air conduction tests**, which stimulate the ear through the air, test the function of the external auditory canal and the middle ear, and the integrity of the inner ear, eighth cranial nerve, and central auditory pathways. **Bone conduction tests** use vibrating tuning forks placed in contact with the head. By bypassing the external auditory canal and middle ear, bone conduction tests can help distinguish problems in the inner ear, eighth cranial nerve, and central auditory pathways.

(3) The Weber and Rinne tuning fork tests distinguish between conductive and sensorineural hearing losses. In **the Rinne test**, air and bone conduction tests are compared. In normal hearing, tones sound louder by air conduction than by bone conduction. In conductive hearing loss, however, the bone-conduction stimulus is perceived as louder. In sensorineural hearing loss, both air and bone conduction sounds are diminished, but the air conduction sound is perceived as louder. The Rinne test is the most sensitive in detecting mild conductive hearing losses if a 256 Hz tuning fork is used. **The Weber test** may be performed using a 256 or a 512 Hz tuning fork. During this test, the stem of a vibrating tuning fork is placed on the head in the midline. If the tone is perceived in the affected ear, this indicates a unilateral conductive hearing loss. In the case of unilateral sensorineural hearing loss, the tone is heard in the unaffected ear instead.

[**Objects**]

Human beings.

[**Materials and Equipments**]

Tuning forks (256 and 512 Hz); cotton ball; rubber hammer.

[**Experimental Procedures**]

(1) For the tuning-fork tests, the examiner, using a rubber reflex hammer on his or her elbow, strikes one tine strongly enough to produce a sound clearly perceived by the examiner at 30 cm.

(2) The Rinne test: In the Rinne test (Figure 9-4), the fork is held 2.5 cm from the

external ear with the tines vibrating toward the ear. The stem of the tuning fork is placed on the mastoid and the subject is asked to indicate when she or he stops hearing the sound. The fork is then held 2. 5 cm from the pinna, and the patient is asked if she or he still hears the sound. If the sound is still audible, air conduction is greater than bone conduction ($AC > BC$ in normal ear); if not, $BC > AC$.

(3) Use a cotton ball to block the external auditory canal (to mimic conductive hearing loss); repeat the Rinne test.

(4) The Weber test (Figure 9-4) may be performed using a 256 or a 512 Hz tuning fork. During this test, the stem of a vibrating tuning fork is placed on the head in the midline. The thickness of the scalp or hair sometimes prevents an accurate response. Ask the patient, "Do you hear this better in the right or the left ear?" If the patient hesitates, then the Weber test shows that sound is not being referred to one ear. If the tone is perceived in the affected ear, this indicates a unilateral conductive hearing loss. In the case of unilateral sensorineural hearing loss, the tone is heard in the unaffected ear instead.

(5) Proper recording of the Rinne test should be "$AC > BC$" or "$BC > AC$" for each ear; for the Weber test, "Weber $\rightarrow$ R" or "Weber $\rightarrow$ L" or "Weber not referred."

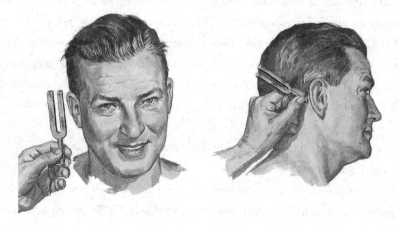

Figure 9-4   Proper positioning of tuning fork tines for air conduction testing(left)and bone conduction (right).

[**Questions**]

1. Compare air conduction and bone conduction.

2. What's the mechanism of conduction deafness and sensorineural hearing loss?

[**Key Words**]

air conduction   bone conduction

(Peng Biwen)

Experiment 29   Cochlear Microphonic Potentials

[Purpose]

To observe the characteristics of the cochlear microphonic potentials and the auditory nerve action potentials and their mutual relations.

[Experimental Principle]

When the cochlea receives sound stimulation, like a microphone, they can transfer the mechanical energy of the acoustic vibration into electricity (electrical signal). This effect of cochleae is called microphonic effect and the potential change is called cochlear microphonic potential (CM). The waveform and frequency of CM correspond to the sound stimulation. Its phase change follows the sound wave and the frequency can be more than 10000 Hz, almost no latency, nor refractory period. There is no adaption and fatigue after a long time of stimulation. When temperature drops, getting anesthesia heavily, or even animals dead within half an hour, CM can also appear. When placing a recording electrode near the inner ear round window of guinea pigs and stimulating with ultrasonic wave, CM occurs followed by it is cochlea nerve action potential, usually 2-3 negative waves (N1, N2 and N3). These negative waves could be the result of the synchronization of nerve fiber action potential and the potential size can reflect the number of excited nerve fibers. After the magnification of the amplifier, cochlear microphonic potential is entered into a computer audio card; we can hear the sound the same as the stimulation sound through computer speakers. This is called microphonic effect.

[Objects]

Guinea pigs (weight: 300~400g, no hearing impairment).

[Materials and Equipments]

Silver ball conventional surgical instruments, bone drill (small size), Physiological signal acquisition processing system RM6240B, recording electrode, 20% urethane, saline at a warm temperature, gauze, cotton ball, injection syringe, operating table, shielded box.

[Experimental Procedures]

(1) Anesthetize guinea pig with 20% urethane (6ml/kg) by intraperitoneal injection.

(2) Cut the hair to make the side of the auricle clean, make an incision on the skin along the posterior superior border of the auricle root, and separate the muscles.

(3) Find the mastoid process of temporal bone (about 1.5cm below the occipital protuberance, 0.5cm rear of external auditory canal opening). Drill a hole with the small bone drill and expand it using tweezers (about 1mm in diameter). The bone is thin and care should be taken when operating to avoid cochlear damage.

(4) Move the animal to the shield box and place it on its side. Curve the recording electrode front slightly; go through the hole into the deep gently to make the silver ball contact

with the round window membrane. Insert the indifferent electrode and grounding electrode into the incision. Connect the recording electrode with physiological signal acquisition processing system channel 1, making the guinea pig grounded. Connect the monitor output to the speaker.

[**Observations**]

(1) Speak, sing and clap near the guinea pig's outer ear, then listen to the speaker.

(2) Observe the cochlear nerve action potential. Increase the stimulator output intensity, and when the screen appears potential fluctuation, adjust the stimulator to display CM, N1 and N2 and identify each other.

(3) Change the intensity of the sound stimulation, and then observe the changes of cochlear microphonic potential and auditory nerve action potential.

(4) Change the phase of the stimulation, and then observe the changes of cochlear microphonic potential and auditory nerve action potential.

[**Notices**]

Avoid the impairment of round window

[**Questions**]

1. Is cochlear microphonic potential retardant?

2. Compare the characteristics of the cochlear microphonic potential and the auditory nerve action potential.

[**Key Words**]

Microphonic effect   cochlear microphonic potential, CM

(Peng Biwen)

Experiment 30   Observation of Nystagmus in Human Body

[**Purpose**]

(1) Observe the nystagmus when a person suddenly stops continuous rotation.

(2) Understand the function of the labyrinth in the internal ear.

[**Principle**]

Nystagmus is a special kind of vestibular reaction when the body has rotatory movement. When a person keeps bowing 30°of his/her head and starts rotating the body along the vertical axis, the hair cells on crista ampullaris in the lateral semicircular canals of both sides will accept different stimulation, causing horizontal nystagmus. When the rotation stops, the hair cells accept the changes of stimulation because the endolymph flows to different directions, causing the second nystagmus with the opposite direction to rotation.

[**Objects**]

Human being.

[**Materials and Equipments**]

A swivel chair.

[**Experimental Procedures**]

The subject sits on a swivel chair, closes the eyes, bow 30°of the head, rotating the chair for 10-15 circles with a velocity of 2 seconds per circle. When the rotation finishes, suddenly stop the chair and have the person open their eyes immediately, recording the movement of the person's eye balls. Observe the nystagmus and distinguish the quick component and slow component of nystagmus. Record the direction and time of duration of quick and slow components.

[**Notices**]

The subject should be protected carefully during the rotation movement to avoid tumbling down or injury.

[**Questions**]

1. How do we judge the direction of nystagmus?

2. What is the relationship of the direction between nystagmus and rotation?

[**Key Words**]

nystagmus

(Wang Yuan)

Chapter 10   The Nervous System

Experiment 31   Analysis of Reflex Arc and Assay of Reflex Time

[**Objective**]

(1) To study the reflex actions in the frog, make a drawing of a complete reflex arc.

(2) Learn how to calculate the reflex time.

[**Principle**]

The term reflex refers to a rapid, automatic response to a stimulus. This action is completed through a reflex arc. A reflex arc consists of a receptor organ, afferent nerve, central nervous system, efferent nerve, and effector organ. During this exercise the behavior of a normal frog will be observed and if any portions of the nervous system are destroyed, the behavior will not be observed.

The time interval from activation of the receptor organ to the response in the effector organ is called reflex time.

[**Object**]

frog.

[**Materials and Equipments**]

Pithing needle, frog board, beakers, filter paper, gauze, stimulating apparatus, 0. 5% H_2SO

[**Methods**]

Destroy the frog's brain from the foramen using the pithing needle to prepare a spinal frog, and suspend the frog so that the limbs hang free.

[**Observe Items**]

1. Assay of Reflex Time

Place one of the hind toes in 0. 5% H_2SO_4. Flexor reflex will be observed. Record the time interval between immersing the toe into the 0. 5% H_2SO_4 and flection of the hind limb. Wash the skin with water and dry it using gauze. Repeat the experiment three times. The mean value of two time intervals is the reflex time.

2. Analysis of Reflex Arc

(1) Place the left toe in 0. 5% H_2SO_4. Flexor reflex will be observed. Wash the skin with water and dry it using filter gauze.

(2) Remove the skin of the left toe below the heel. Repeat step 1.

(3) Place the right toe in 0.5% H_2SO_4. Flexor reflex will be observed. Wash the skin with water and dry it using filter gauze.

(4) Isolate and cut the right Sciatic nerve, placing the right toe in 0.5% H_2SO_4. Observe the response of left and right hind legs.

(5) Stimulate (2V, 0.2ms, 20Hz) the central end of the right sciatic nerve, observing the response of left and right hind legs.

(6) Stimulate (2V, 0.2ms, 20Hz) the periphery of the right sciatic nerve, observing the response of left and right hind legs.

(7) Destroy the spinal cord with pithing needle, repeat step 3.

[**Points of Attention**]

1. Make sure to destroy the brain completely in order to avoid autonomic activities.

2. Make sure that the toe is immersed in 0.5% H_2SO_4 to the same extent and don't immerse too much.

3. Once the reflex occurs, wash the skin with water quickly and dry it using gauze to avoid the skin injury.

[**Question**]

1. What factors influence the length of reflex time?

2. In this experiment, what parts does the flexor reflex arc consist of? In each step, which part has been destroyed?

[**Key Words**]

reflex arc   reflex action   reflex time

(Shi Junzhi)

Experiment 32   Decerebrate Rigidity

[**Purpose**]

To observe the postural control by brain stem.

[**Principle**]

Posture control relies on the variation of muscle tension. The central nervous system has some areas that facilitate and inhibit the stretch reflexes to regulate the muscle tension. When the brain stem is transected between the superior and inferior colliculus, the balance of facilitator and inhibitory impulses shifts toward facilitation. In experimental animals under this condition, the most prominent finding is marked spasticity of the body musculature called decerebrate rigidity. In decerebrate posturing, the head and back are arched backward, and the limbs are rigidly extended.

[Object]

rabbit.

[Materials and Equipments]

20% Urethane, 0. 9% saline, rongeur, bone drill, cotton, gauze and rabbit surgical instrument kit.

[Methods]

1. Anesthesia

Weigh the rabbit and intravenously inject 20% Urethane at the dose of 0. 5-0. 8g/kg to anesthetize the rabbit.

2. Operation

(1) Fix the rabbit on the head frame and shear the hair on the vertex of the head.

(2) Incise the skin along the midline from glabella to occipital, and dissect the subcutaneous tissue and muscle to expose the skull.

(3) Drill a hole in the parietal bone with the bone drill

(4) Enlarge the hole with the rongeur. After opening the unilateral skull, insert the blade handle into the space between the sagittal sinus and skull to separate the sagittal sinus from skull. Remove the contralateral skull with the rongeur until bilateral cerebral hemispheres are exposed. Incise the dura covering on the surface of cerebral cortex.

(5) Dissect the occipital lobe from the trailing edge of the cerebral hemispheres to expose superior and inferior colliculus. Insert the blade between superior and inferior colliculus toward mandible angle to transect the brain stem.

[Observing Items]

Observe the posture change of the limbs, neck, back and tail. If the posture change is not obvious, lift the rabbit and vibrate it to enhance the extensor stretch reflex.

[Points of Attention]

(1) Too deep of anesthesia can weaken the decerebrate rigidity.

(2) Don't destroy the sagittal sinus while enlarging the hole in the skull.

(3) Transect the brain stem at the precise position. Transection at lower position may destroy the medulla to initiate breath stopping, whereas transection at a higher position may fail to induce decerebrate rigidity.

[Questions]

Why is the decerebrate rigidity initiated following brain stem transection?

[Key Words]

decerebrate rigidity

(Wang Zefen)

Experiment 33   Functional Localization of Cerebral Motor Cortex

[**Purpose**]

　　(1) To observe the motor responses induced by electrical stimulation of cortical motor cortex.

　　(2) To apprehend the characteristic of somatic movement control by cortical motor areas.

[**Principle**]

　　The motor cortex controls body movements. Motor signals initiated from the motor cortex are transmitted to the spinal cord and motor nuclei of the cranial nerves through pyramidal system and extrapyramidal system. These motor neurons, in turn, send specific control signals to the skeletal muscles. By means of electrical stimulation in patients undergoing neurosurgical operations, a topographical representation of the various muscle areas of the body in the motor cortex have been mapped. The representation area in the motor cortex is proportionate in size to the skill with which the part is used. This topographical organization in human beings is far more developed than in rodents such as the rat and rabbit.

[**Object**]

　　rabbit (weight 2-2. 5kg).

[**Materials and Equipments**]

　　20% urethane, 0. 9% saline, liquid paraffin, BL-420E bio-signal recording system, rongeur, bone drill, cotton, stimulation electrode and rabbit surgical instrument kit.

[**Methods**]

1. Anesthesia

Intravenously inject 20% Urethane at the dose of 0. 8-1. 0 g/kg to anesthetize the rabbit.

2. Operation

　　(1) Fix the rabbit on the head frame and shear the hair on the vertex of the head.

　　(2) Incise the skin along the midline from glabella to occipital, and dissect the subcutaneous tissue and muscle to expose the cranial bone.

　　(3) Drill a hole in the parietal bone with the bone drill(Figure 10-1).

　　(4) Enlarge the hole with the rongeur. After opening the unilateral skull, insert blade handle into the space between sagittal sinus and skull to separate sagittal sinus from skull. Remove the contralateral skull with the rongeur until bilateral cerebral hemispheres are exposed.

　　(5) Incise the dura covering on the surface of cerebral cortex. Drop liquid paraffin (37℃) on the surface of cerebral cortex to protect the brain.

3. Observing Items

　　Electrically stimulate (10-20V, 0. 2ms, 20Hz) the various areas of cortical surface in turn and observe the motor responses. Compare the results with the following representation map (Figure 10-2).

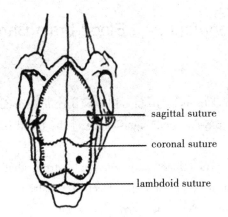

Figure 10-1   Surgical operation area on the vertex of rabbit

(The black dot represents the position where the hole is drilled)

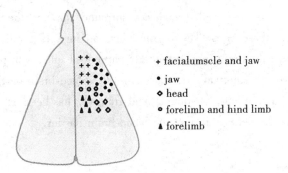

Figure 10-2   Motor functional areas of the rabbit cerebral cortex

[**Points of Attention**]

　　(1) Deep anesthesia can weaken the motor responses to electrical stimulation.

　　(2) Carefully enlarge the hole in the skull and avoid injuring the sagittal sinus.

　　(3) Protect the cerebral cortex during the surgical operation.

[**Questions**]

　　Describe the characteristics of motor controlling by the motor cortex.

[**Key Words**]

　　cerebral cortex

(Wang Zefen)

Experiment 34   Blood-brain Barrier

[**Purpose**]

(1) To learn the method to measure blood-brain barrier permeability.

(2) To apprehend the physiological significance of the blood-brain barrier.

[**Principle**]

Blood-brain barrier is a functional and structural barrier that controls the extracellular neuronal environment within the brain and spinal cord by restricting the passage of substances from the bloodstream into the CNS. The barrier is permeable to water, CO_2, O_2 and lipid-soluble molecules, but almost impermeable to non-lipid soluble large molecules. The "barrier" predominantly results from the particular arrangement of capillary endothelial cells. The endothelial cells are stitched together by tight junctions and surrounded by a basement membrane. Astrocytic processes called end-feet surround the endothelial cells and provide biochemical support to those cells. The barrier plays an important role to maintain a stable environment and protect the brain from potentially harmful chemicals in the blood circulation.

Trypan blue, a dye that normally does not cross the blood-brain barrier because of its size (MW 916 Da) and hydrophilicity (4 sulfonic acid groups), has been extensively used as a test reagent to demonstrate the permeability of the blood-brain barrier.

[**Objects**]

Mouse.

[**Materials and Equipments**]

diethyl ether, 1 ml syringe, needle, scissor, and 1% trypan blue.

[**Method**]

(1) Anesthetize the mouse by inhalation of ether.

(2) Intraperitoneally inject 1ml of 1% trypan blue, or intravenously inject 0. 5ml of 1% trypan blue.

(3) Observe the color change of the eye and mouth. Kill the mouse when the eyes and mouth become blue and dissect the whole body. Observe the color of skin, lung, liver, guts, brain, and spinal cord, and compare them with corresponding organs in normal mouse.

[**Questions**]

1. Why is the color in brain and spinal cord different from other organs after trypan blue injection?

2. What is the physiological significance of blood-brain barrier?

[**Key Words**]

blood-brain barrier

(Wang Zefen)

Experiment 35   The Effect of One Side Cerebellum Damage on Body Movement

[**Purpose**]

To observe the abnormal motor activity induced by cerebellum injury.

[**Principle**]

Cerebellum is also essential for controlling of normal motor function. Cerebellum does not initiate movement, but it plays major roles in coordination, precision, and accurate timing of motor activities. Functionally, the cerebellum is divided into three parts. ①Vestibulocerebellum functions in association with the brain stem and spinal cord to control equilibrium and postural movements. ②Spinocerebellum provided smooth and coordinate movements by continuous input from the motor cortex and peripheral parts of the body. ③Cerebrocerebellum is associated with planning, sequencing, and timing of complex movements. Cerebellar damage does not cause paralysis of any muscles, but instead produces disorders in fine movement, equilibrium and posture, such as ataxia.

[**Object**]

mouse.

[**Materials and Equipments**]

Ether, cotton, scissors, forceps, needle.

[**Methods**]

1. Anesthesia

Anesthetize the mouse by ether inhalation.

2. Operation

(1) Incise the skin along the midline of the vertex to occipital, and dissect the subcutaneous tissue and muscle to expose the cranial bone.

(2) Insert a needle into one side of the cerebellum and destroy it by vibrating the needle several times in fore and aft direction. Remove the needle and stop bleeding by pressure with cotton. Coordinates relative to lambdoid suture and the surface of the brain (posterior, mediolateral, and dorsoventral, respectively) is 1, 2, 3 mm for insert (Figure 10-3).

[**Observing Items**]

After the mouse is awake, observe the change in equilibrium and posture movements. Observe whether the mouse with cerebellum injury exhibits uncoordinated movement or not.

[**Points of Attention**]

(1) The depth of insert is 3mm. Too deep of injury may destroy the medulla.

(2) If the symptom is not obvious, destroy the cerebellum again from the same position.

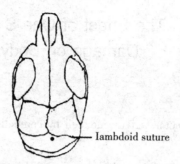

Iambdoid suture

Figure 10-3   The position to destroy the cerebellum in mouse
(the black dot indicates the point to insert the needle)

[**Questions**]

What is the change of somatic movement and body equilibrium in the mouse following injury of one side cerebellum?

[**Key Words**]

cerebellum injury

(Wang Zefen)

Experiment 36   Biceps Reflex

[**Purpose**]

Study the methods to test biceps reflex.

[**Principle**]

Reflexes are the most objective part of the neurologic examination and they are very helpful in determining the level of damage to the nervous system. Biceps reflex is a common reflex test that examines the function of the C5 reflex arc and the C6 reflex arc.

[**Object**]

human beings.

[**Equipments**]

Tendon hammer.

[**Experimental Procedures**]

(1) Identify the location of the biceps tendon. To do this, have the patient flex at the elbow while you observe and palpate the antecubital fossa. The tendon will look and feel like a thick cord.

(2) Let the patient rest the arm in the patient's lap, forming an angle of slightly more than 90 degrees at the elbow. Make sure that the bicep muscle is completely relaxed.

(3) It may be difficult to direct your hammer strike such that the force is transmitted directly on to the biceps tendon, and not dissipated amongst the rest of the soft tissue in the area. Place your index or middle fingers firmly against the tendon and strike them with the hammer.

(4) Make sure that the patient's sleeve is rolled up so that you can directly observe the muscle as well as watch the lower arm for movement. A normal response will cause the biceps to contract, drawing the lower arm upwards.

[Notices]

keep the subject relaxed.

[Key Words]

biceps reflex

(Zhang Xianrong)

Experiment 37　　Knee Jerk Reflex

[Principle]

The knee jerk reflex, also called patellar reflex, is when a tendon above the kneecap is tapped with a reflex hammer, which causes the whole leg to involuntarily jerk. Striking the patellar ligament with a reflex hammer just below the patella stretches the muscle spindle in the quadriceps muscle. This produces a signal which travels back to the spinal cord. From there, an alpha-motor neuron conducts an efferent impulse back to the quadriceps femoris muscle, triggering contraction. This contraction, coordinated with the relaxation of the antagonistic flexor hamstring muscle causes the leg to kick. Legs that do not jerk at all or that jerk continuously after being tapped are considered abnormal.

The patellar reflex is a clinical and classic example of the monosynaptic reflex because there is only one synapse in the circuit needed to complete the reflex.

[Experimental Procedures]

(1) Have a partner sit with his or her legs crossed so that the leg can swing freely.

(2) Tap the knee at a spot just below the kneecap (Figure 10-4). The leg will jerk immediately if you hit the right place.

[Subject]

human beings.

[Materials and Equipments]

rubber hammer.

[Notices]

Keep the subject relaxed.

[**Key Words**]

knee jerk feflex

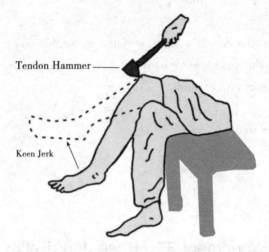

Tendon Hammer

Keen Jerk

Figure 10-4   Knee jerk reflex

(Wang Zefen)

Experiment 38   Achilles Tendon Reflex

[**Purpose**]

to learn how to detect achilles tendon reflex and know the mechanism of human spinal reflex.

[**Principle**]

Achilles tendon reflex is also called ankle jerk, which is a deep monosynaptic stretch reflex. It can be initiated tapping the Achilles tendon in the dorsi-flexed status. The positive response appears the jerking of the foot toward its plantar surface.

[**Subject**]

human being.

[**Material**]

rubber hammer.

[**Method**]

(1) Keep subject in supine position and knee joint in abduction

(2) Hold one foot and make itslightly dorsi-flexed, striking the Achilles tendon lightly with a rubber hammer.

(3) Hold the other foot, and repeat step(2).

[**Item**]

observe the response.

[**Notice**]

(1) keep the subject relaxed;

(2) keep the striking site precise.

[**Question**]

What are the similar and different points between tendon reflex and muscle tonus?

[**Key Words**]

achilles tendon reflex

(Chen Taoxiang)

序　言

1. 概述

生理学是一门实验性极强的科学。最早从事生理学研究的科学家是 17 世纪英国的著名医生 William Harvey，他采用活体解剖的方法在动物体上进行研究，同时通过观察人体现象，才得出血液循环的正确结论。1628 年 William Harvey 出版了《心血运动论》。所以生理学这门学科是建立在实验和观察基础上的，充分说明了生理学实验对生理学创立和发展的重要作用。因此国内外生理学家无不重视生理学实验课，因为一个只能记忆生理学概念而不会动手的人，是不可能对实验性学科做出贡献的。

(1) 生理实验教学的性质、任务和目的

通过实验获得知识的科学属于实验科学。生理医学知识来源于科学实验，是一门实践性很强的实验科学。17 世纪初，英国 William Harvey 首先在动物身上用活体解剖和科学实验的方法研究了血液循环，证明心脏是循环系统的中心，血液由心脏射入动脉，再由静脉回流入心，不断循环。1628 年，Harvey 的著作《心与血的运动》出版，是历史上第一本基本实验证据的生理学著作，标志着生理学成为一门独立的学科。因此，科学实验创立和发展了生理学理论，是研究生理学的基本方法。要真正学好生理学，必须同时重视理论课和实验课的学习，两者相辅相成，不可分割。

开设生理学实验教学课程，目的在于：①通过实验使学生逐步掌握生理学实验的基本操作技术，了解生理学实验设计的基本原则，进一步了解获得生理学知识的方法，验证和巩固生理学的某些基本理论。②通过实验使学生逐步提高对实验中各种生理现象的观察能力、分析能力、独立思考和独立解决问题的能力。③学习必需的实验技术方法，通过这些方法引发出自然状态下单凭感官观察不到的现象，引导学生观察实验现象，通过思考探寻现象与本质的联系，实现深化认识已知，探索未知，培养学生动脑、动手的能力和探索创新的精神。④在实验过程中，逐步培养学生在科学工作中严肃的态度、严格的要求、严格的方法和严谨的作风。

(2) 生理学实验及其方法

生理学实验即是利用一定的仪器设备和方法，人为地控制某些因素以再现动物机体的某些生命活动过程，或将一些感官难以观察到的内在的、迅速而微小变化着的生命活动展现、记录下来，便于人们观察、分析和研究。

因为生理学是研究动物机体生命活动(机能)及其规律的一门学科，因此生理学实验的对象一般都是机能正常的"活体"，而且这种"活体"的特征在动物机体的整体、器

官及细胞等不同水平上有不同的表现形式。

根据动物的组织器官是在整体条件下进行实验，还是将其解剖取下置于人工环境条件下进行实验，一般可将生理学实验的方法分为在体(in vivo)实验方法和离体(ex vivo)实验方法，也可分为急性动物实验和慢性动物实验。

1)急性动物实验

选择动物的整体或离体标本，或先给动物机体造成损伤，然后在短期间内观察机体或器官所发生的变化。通常是将动物固定，在局麻或全身麻醉下进行实验。按实验需要可分离出血管或神经，打开胸腔或腹腔，记录各器官的机能活动，如描记血压、呼吸等。这是教学实验中常用的方法，可在短时间内获得实验结果，较易阐明一些现象和理论。一般又可分急性整体动物实验和急性离体实验。

①急性整体动物实验。急性整体动物实验是在整体水平上主要研究心血管、呼吸、泌尿和消化功能及其神经体液调节的实验方法。它是生理学实验中常用的实验方法，也是近似生理情况下进行的一种实验方法。这种方法比较简单，易于控制条件，有利于观察器官间的具体关系和分析某一器官功能活动的过程与特点。但是，由于动物失去知觉，破坏了机体与外界的相互作用，与正常生理情况下的功能活动仍有差别。另外，整体的实验受到体内神经体液调节和各种复杂因素的干扰，较难深入了解药物作用的本质和各种变化的细节与内在规律。要分析药物作用机理时还需结合离体实验，两者取长补短、相互补充。

急性整体动物实验常用的方法有：血压测定法、呼吸运动描记法和泌尿、消化功能测定法等。

②急性离体实验。离体实验是根据实验目的和对象的需要，将所需的动物器官或组织按照一定的程序从动物机体上分离下来，置于人工环境中，设法在短时间内保持它的生理功能而进行研究的一种实验方法。此种方法的优点在于能摒弃组织或器官在体内受到多种生理因素的综合作用，从而能比较明确地确定某种因素与特定生理反应的关系。但由于离体实验的实验对象已去除了整体时中枢神经的控制，所以离体实验得出的结论还不能直接推广至整体时的情况。因此，对于一种机理的论证，必须结合整体实验结果加以阐明。离体器官、组织实验常用的方法有离体心脏、离体骨骼肌、离体平滑肌实验法等。

2)慢性动物实验

慢性动物实验是使动物处于清醒状态下，观察动物整体活动或某一器官对于体内情况或外界条件变化时的反应。在做慢性实验前，首先在无菌条件下，给动物施行一定的实验手术，根据实验目的要求，对动物进行一定的处理，如导出或去除某个器官，或埋入某种电极或药物，待其恢复接近正常生活状态，再观察所暴露器官的某些功能或摘除、破坏某器官后产生的生理功能紊乱等现象。

慢性实验的最大优点是保持了实验动物机体的完整及其与外界环境的统一性，动物处于比较接近自然的状态。因此，所观察到的实验结果比较符合于客观实际，也比较正确可靠，但由于观察时间长，对实验设备和技术要求高，影响因素较多，因而难度较大。故在生理学实验教学中较少采用，而广泛应用于研究工作中。

2. 教学要求和实验室守则

根据生理学实验课的要求和提高实验课教学质量的需要，要求教师和学生共同努力。因此，实验课的要求包括实验前、实验过程中和实验后的操作以及对教师和学生两个方面。

(1) 实验前

①集体备课。生理学实验是在生命机体上进行的，易受各方面因素的制约和影响，实验前进行集体备课是保证实验顺利完成的基本条件。集体备课应在主管教师的统一指导下进行，负责实验的人员(包括教师、研究生、实验技术人员)全部参加。在备课中，明确实验的目的要求、统一实验的方法步骤、规定实验的项目和内容。并要求教师熟练掌握。

②学生必须仔细预习实验指导。了解实验的目的要求、基本原理以及简要的操作步骤。实验课开始后，教师若发现学生未预习，应令其停止实验，待其预习后再进行。

③学生应复习有关理论，以便提高实验过程中的主动性和效率，并进一步巩固有关理论知识。

(2) 实验过程中

①教师应严格要求学生，对必须学会的基本操作技术应一丝不苟，培养学生科学的素养和分析问题、解决问题的能力。

②学生应认真、仔细地进行各项操作，观察实验中出现的各种现象，如实地随时加以记录，并对引起各种生理现象的原因、意义进行分析与思考。

③实验器材要安放整齐，布局合理，便于操作。要保持清洁卫生，随时清除污物。实验桌上不得放置与实验无关的物品。

④爱护仪器与实验动物，注意节约各种实验材料。公用物品在使用完毕后应放回原处，以免影响别人使用。

⑤保持实验室安静，不得嬉笑与高声谈话，以免影响别人做实验。

⑥遵守实验室规则，注意实验小组内的团结、配合与分工协作。

(3) 实验后

①学生应将实验用具整理就绪，放回原处。所用手术器械必须擦洗干净。实验用具如有损坏或缺少，应即报告指导教师。做好实验室的清洁卫生工作。

②妥善处理实验动物，若实验结束后动物尚未死亡，应在教师指导下处死，而后放于指定地点。

③整理实验记录，认真书写、及时交实验报告。

④教师应认真批改实验报告。若发现不符合要求的实验报告，应指明问题，退回重写。

(4) 生理实验课教学对学生的要求

学生是学习的主体，只有领会课程的总体目标和每一次实验的目的，才能主动、高效地学习。本教程总论各章内容学生必须认真自学。每次实验课前必须认真做好预习和准备，内容主要包括：实验目的和原理、相关的理论知识和背景、所用仪器的使用方法及参数设置、动物手术操作方法、需要观察的指标及意义、预测各项实验处理的反应、所用试剂溶液的成分及配制方法、思考题和作业题中涉及的相关内容等。只有做到心中有数，有备而来，才能达到实验教学的目的。

实验过程中要按程序正确操作、善于观察、认真记录、勤于思考。通过思考去剖析实验中引发的现象，做到观察与思考互为补充、相得益彰，不仅可深化认识已知，也将有所发现、有所创新，从而激发求知欲和学习兴趣。为能真正鼓励学生开发并表达自己的想法，实现创造力教学的理念，本教程在每个实验项目后面提供了一些需要进一步探索的问题，以激发学生进一步去思考。学生也可选择一些问题，按照实验设计要求书写实验设计书，经指导老师修改后，提出书面申请，到开放性实验室实施探索性实验。

搞好同学之间的协作，提倡多讨论问题，相互启发，相互学习，相互帮助，共同提高，培养这种团队精神和品德是实验教学的目标之一。

实验后，要按规定整理实验器具和处理实验动物，做好实验室的清洁卫生工作。学生应及时整理实验记录，认真撰写实验报告，按时交给教师批阅。

（5）生理实验课教学对教师的要求

教师不仅应该具备所涉学科的基本知识和新的信息，还应牢固树立教书育人的观念和新的教学理念，充满激情，善于引导学生观察、思考、开拓思路，鼓励学生质疑、表达想法、积极动手，让学生享受实验科学的无穷乐趣，激发求知欲和学习兴趣。每次实验课教师应充分备课，按照教学大纲要求讲授相关内容，提问并记录成绩。在实验中，教师要注重培养学生的协作和团队精神。在总结实验时，教师应注重引导学生如何对实验结果进行整理、推理分析，导出科学的结论，实现深化认识已知，探索未知的教学目的。教师应鼓励学生参与自己开展的科研工作，借以培养学生的科研能力。

（6）实验室守则

生理学实验课的目的是通过实验使学生逐步掌握生理学实验的基本操作技术，了解生理学实验设计的基本原则，进一步了解获得生理学知识的方法，验证和巩固生理学的某些基本理论。通过实验使学生逐步提高对实验中各种生理现象的观察能力、分析能力、独立思考和独立解决问题的能力。在实验过程中，逐步培养学生在科学工作中严肃认真的态度、严格的要求、严格的方法和严谨的作风。

为了提高实验课的教学质量，学生必须仔细预习实验指导，了解实验的目和要求、基本原理以及简要的操作步骤。实验课开始后，教师如发现学生未预习，应令其停止实验，待其预习后再进行。学生应认真、仔细地进行各项操作，观察实验中出现的各种现象，如实地随时加以记录，并对引起各种生理现象的原因、意义进行分析与思考。每个学生应严格遵守以下实验室规则：

①遵守学习纪律，准时上、下课。实验期间不得借故外出或早退。特殊情况下，应向教师请假。

②必须严肃认真地进行实验操作、观察实验结果。实验期间要保持安静，不得进行任何与实验无关的活动。

③实验所得数据及实验记录需经教师审核，否则不得结束实验。

④各组的仪器和用品，由本组使用，不得与别组调换，以免引起混乱。若遇仪器损坏或丢失，应报请教师处理。

⑤爱护公共财物，注意节约各种实验用品。实验动物按组发给，如需补充使用，须经教师同意才能补领。

⑥保持实验室清洁整齐，随时清除污物。实验完毕后，应将实验器材、用品收拾妥当，将手术器械擦洗干净，清点数量，放回原处。经教师检查后才能离开实验室。

3. 实验报告的书写方法

写实验报告是生理学实验课的基本训练之一，应以科学的态度认真、严肃地对待，以便为日后撰写科学论文打下良好的基础。为帮助学生书写报告，现将其格式、内容和要求作一简要说明。

(1)实验结束后，均需根据指导教师的要求，每人写一份实验报告，并按时完成，及对送交指导教师评阅。

(2)实验报告的格式与内容。

①注明姓名、专业、组别、日期。

②实验序号及题目。

③实验目的要求。

④实验方法：应根据教师的具体要求写。一般情况下或重复使用的方法可作简要说明。

⑤实验结果：实验结果是实验报告的重要部分，应将实验过程中所观察或记录到的生理效应忠实地、正确地记述和说明。结果部分常需用实验记录，这就需要将实验记录进行合理地加工与剪贴，并加图号、图注及必要的文字说明。不得将原始记录原封不动地附在报告上，凡属定量的测量资料，例如快慢、轻重、长短、多少等，均应以正确的单位和数值严格地写在报告上。为了说明实验的可靠性，有些实验结果需要作统计学处理，求出均数、标准差以及显著性检验。

⑥实验结果的处理及表示：实验结果包括实验过程中观察到的现象、记录曲线、数据等，这些结果一般称为原始资料。原始资料分为两大类：一类是计量资料，另一类为计数资料，实验者务必分清这两类资料的区别。凡属曲线记录的实验，应对曲线进行整理，具体方法参见附录三。为了便于说明和比较，有些实验结果可以列表或绘图表示。绘制棒状图和坐标图的方法、要求、注意事项参见附录四。

⑦讨论与结论：讨论是根据所学的理论知识，对实验结果进行科学地分析和解释，并判断实验结果是否是预期的。如果出现非预期的结果，应分析其可能的原因。讨论是实验报告的核心部分，可以帮助学生提高独立思考和分析问题的能力。不应盲目抄袭书本，应提倡学生根据自己的实验结果提出创造性的见解和认识，但必须是严肃认真、有科学依据的。结论是从实验结果和讨论中归纳出一般的概括性的判断，也就是这一实验所验证的基本概念、原则或理论的简明总结。结论的书写应该是简明扼要的。

（彭碧文）

第1章 RM6240 生物信号记录系统

1.1 系统特点

RM6240 生理信号采集处理系统(包括 RM6240B 和 RM6240C 两种型号)是成都仪器厂研制的新一代医学实验设备。RM6240 有 EPP(并口机型)和 USB 两种类型接口。系统采用 12 位 A/D 转换器,采样频率在实时显示曲线、动态存盘情况下高达 100kHz(并口机型)或 200kHz(PCI 高速机型)。

系统具有多通道多功能全程控放大器:通过模式选择,每一通道的放大器均可作为生物电放大器、血压放大器、桥式放大器使用,还可作为肺量计(配接流量换能器)、温度计(配接温度换能器)、pH 计(配接 pH 放大器)。另外,还具备记滴、监听、全隔离程控刺激器。也可在任意通道对各通道动态地进行微分、积分、频谱分析及相关分析等数据处理。

系统由硬件和软件(RM6240 生理信号采集处理系统)两部分组成。硬件包括外置程控放大器、数据采集板、数据线及各种信号输入输出线。面板上设置有外接信号输入插座、刺激器输出插座、记滴及监听插座。

1.2 仪器面板

(1)通道输入接口。通道是模拟信号输入、处理放大、转换成数字信号并显示记录的物理通路,该系统可同时处理放大和记录 4 路信号。

(2)刺激输出接口。通过刺激连线可输出刺激电压或电流,刺激波形为方波。

(3)受滴器输入接口。将此接口与受滴器相连,可用于记录液体的滴数。该接口也可用于外触发信号输入。

(4)监听输出接口。将此接口与音箱连接,可监听指定通道信号的声音。

1.3 窗口界面

RM6240 软件窗口界面可划分为 6 个功能区:

（1）菜单栏。位于界面顶端，可显示顶层菜单项。选择其中的一项即可弹出下拉式子菜单。

（2）工具条。工具条位于菜单栏的下方。工具条提供菜单栏中最常用指令的快捷按钮，用鼠标直接点击即可激活相应功能。

（3）参数控制区。参数控制区位于窗口界面的右侧。每个通道参数区均具备多项功能显示，包括通道模式、扫描速度、灵敏度、时间常数、滤波频率和导联。用鼠标点击相应功能键即可调节各通道的实验参数。

（4）数据显示区。数据显示区位于窗口界面的中间主体区域，实验数据以波形的形式显示于该区域。

（5）标尺及处理区。该区域位于窗口界面的左侧，显示各通道的通道号及相应信号的标尺。选择该区域的"处理"按钮，弹出菜单栏中可显示通道定标、标记显示、分析测量和数据处理等功能选项。

（6）刺激器。程控刺激器为弹出式浮动窗口，可通过每一参数项右边的上下箭头调节窗口对话框中的参数设置。

1.4　基 本 功 能

1.4.1　仪器参数

1. 仪器参数的快捷设置方法

大多数实验项目的参数已预先设置。启动系统软件后，在"实验"菜单栏中选择所需进行的实验项目，系统即自动将仪器参数设置为该实验项目所需状态。

2. 放大器的参数设置

（1）通道模式选择：点击"通道模式"，在下拉菜单中选择记录信号的形式。

（2）仪器的带通设置。

①时间常数：调节放大器的低频滤波的程度，如 1s，0.1s，0.01s 和 0.001s 分别对应放大器的下限截至频率为 0.16Hz，1.6Hz，16Hz 和 160Hz。

②滤波频率：调节放大器的高频滤波。当所记录信号有效成分频率较低时，应选择低滤波频率，以滤除高频干扰。

（3）采样频率：采用频率是指系统采集数据的频率，其范围为 1Hz～100kHz。在实验过程中，应根据所记录信号的频率选择合适的采样频率，信号频率高则选择高采样频率，信号频率低则选择低采样频率。

（4）灵敏度：该参数用于选择放大器的放大倍数。当所观察信号过大或过小时，可相应地减小或提高灵敏度，从而调整信号显示区中的信号幅度以便观察和分析。

1.4.2 信号记录

1. 信号记录快捷按钮
四个按钮的功能分别是：

(1)示波按钮：启动"示波"按钮，可将记录的信号实时动态地显示在"信号显示记录区"内。在示波状态下，可进行系统参数、采样频率调节等，但不能保存数据。

(2)记录按钮：启动"记录"按钮，可将所记录的信号实时动态显示在"信号显示记录区"，同时能在硬盘中保存相应信号的数据。

(3)暂停按钮：点击"暂停"按钮，信号停止并显示存盘。若再点击"记录"按钮，信号继续显示并存盘于同一页内。

(4)停止按钮：点击"停止"按钮，信号停止并显示存盘。若再次点击"记录"按钮，信号将换页显示和存盘(可用键盘上的"Page Up"和"Page Down"键显示各记录页)。

2. 同步触发记录
打开刺激器窗口，选中"触发同步"功能。点击"开始刺激"按钮即可记录信号，信号从左至右显示一"屏"。信号显示的"屏"数由"重复"次数决定。

1.4.3 刺激器功能及设置

当实验项目需要对实验对象进行刺激时，可打开刺激器，选择刺激方式，调节刺激参数。

1. 功能选项
(1)同步触发：当选择同步触发时，系统采集信号和刺激器发出的刺激脉冲将同步进行，每发一次刺激，系统采集并显示一屏波形。

(2)记录当前波形：系统以子文件形式保持当前屏幕波形。每点击一次该键，即保存一屏波形，子文件逐一保存。可通过键盘上的"Page Up"和"Page Down"键依次查看各子文件中的实验波形。

(3)不叠加：每发一次刺激，显示一屏最新采集的原始波形。

(4)叠平均：每发一次刺激，以当前采集的一屏波形和此前同步采集的所有波形叠加平均后再显示在屏幕上。

(5)叠累积：以当前采集的一屏波形和此前同步采集的波形叠加后再显示在屏幕上。

(6)开始刺激：点击该按钮，刺激器将按设定的方式和刺激参数发出刺激脉冲。

(7)停止刺激：点击该按钮，刺激器将停止发出脉冲刺激。

2. 刺激参数
刺激器输出的刺激脉冲的波形是方波，基本参数如下：

(1)刺激强度：指输出脉冲的电压或电流的强度。脉冲电压范围为 $0 \sim 50V$，脉冲电流范围为 $0 \sim 10mA$。

（2）刺激波宽：指单个脉冲（方波）高电平的持续时间，即刺激的持续时间，波宽可在 0.1~1000ms 调节。

（3）刺激波间隔：指在连续脉冲刺激下，刺激脉冲之间的时间间隔，波间隔可调节范围为 0.1~1000ms。波间隔与波宽之和的倒数可理解为刺激频率，调节范围为 1~3000Hz。

（4）主周期：刺激器以周期为时间单位输出序列脉冲。一个主周期内，刺激脉冲可以是一个、数个，甚至数百个，波间隔可因实验需求设定。"周期数"是指以主周期为单位序列脉冲的循环输出次数。主周期、延迟、波宽、波间隔和脉冲数设置要符合：主周期(s)>延时(s)+[波宽(s)+波间隔(s)]×脉冲数。

（5）脉冲数：指刺激器在设定的时间内发出刺激脉冲的个数。

（6）延迟：指从刺激器启动到刺激脉冲输出的延搁时间。在触发同步记录时，延迟可用来调节反应信号在屏幕上的水平位置。

3. 输出方式

刺激器有恒压（电压）和恒流（电流）两种输出方式。恒压输出方式有正电压和负电压两种脉冲，恒流输出方式也有正电流和负电流两种脉冲。

4. 刺激模式

按一定的主周期、脉冲数和波间隔等参数可将刺激脉冲编制成某种特定脉冲序列，这种特定脉冲序列称为刺激模式。该仪器基本的刺激模式可适用各种实验的需要，具体如下：

（1）单刺激：指在一个主周期内输出一个刺激脉冲，可调节参数有强度、波宽、延时、主周期和重复次数。该刺激模式可采用同步触发的方式记录信号，常用于神经干动作电位、骨骼肌单收缩、期前收缩和诱发电位等实验。

（2）连续单刺激：连续单刺激是指主周期为 1s，无限循环的连续刺激，在一个主周期内输出的脉冲数等于频率，且脉冲的波间隔相等。该刺激模式常用于刺激减压神经、迷走神经，或观察刺激频率对骨骼肌收缩的影响实验。

（3）双刺激：指在一个主周期内输出两个刺激脉冲，可调节参数有强度、波宽、延时、波间隔、主周期和重复次数。该刺激模式可采用同步触发的方式记录信号，常用于骨骼肌收缩、不应期测定等实验。

（4）串单刺激：指在一个主周期内输出序列刺激脉冲，序列脉冲的脉冲数为 3~999 个，可调节参数有强度、波宽、延时、波间隔、主周期、脉冲数和重复次数。该刺激模式可采用同步触发的方式记录，常用于刺激减压神经、迷走神经，或观察刺激频率对骨骼肌收缩的影响实验。

（5）定时刺激：指在设定的刺激持续时间内，刺激脉冲按设定的频率输出，可调节参数有延时、波宽、幅度、刺激时间、频率、主周期和重复次数。该刺激模式常用于观察同一刺激时间内，不同刺激频率的刺激效果，如刺激减压神经、迷走神经，或观察刺激频率对骨骼肌收缩的影响实验。

（6）强度递增：指刺激强度从初始强度开始按一定增量自动递增发出刺激脉冲。选定该方式后，需确定初始刺激参数、组间延时及各组间的强度增量。该刺激模式常用于刺激强度与反应的测定实验。

(7)频率递增：指刺激频率从初始频率开始按一定增量自动递增发出刺激脉冲。选定该刺激方式后，需确定初始刺激参数、组间延时及各组间的频率增量。该刺激模式常用于刺激频率与反应的测定实验。

(8)波宽递增：指刺激波宽从初始波宽开始按一定增量自动递增发出刺激脉冲。选择该方式后，需确定初始刺激参数、组间延时及波宽增量。该刺激模式常用于基强度和时值的测定实验。

(9)串双刺激：指由两个刺激脉冲组成一个脉冲组，在一个主周期内可输出数个至数百个脉冲组，可调节参数有强度、波宽、延时、波间隔、频率、组数、主周期和重复次数。

(10)连续双刺激：连续双刺激与串双刺激作用基本相同，主周期内的脉冲组数用频率表示。

(11)高级功能：在高级功能窗口下，可根据需要将不同主周期、强度、波间隔和脉冲数等刺激模式组成刺激序列，构成程控刺激器。

(张先荣)

第 2 章　生理学实验基本操作技术

2.1　实验动物的基本知识

2.1.1　实验动物分类

实验动物必须具有明确的生物学特性和清楚的遗传背景，并且其所携带的微生物、寄生虫须经过严格控制。

1. 实验动物按遗传学原理分类

（1）近交系动物（inbred strains of animals），即纯系动物，按血缘关系采用至少 20 代近亲交配如兄妹交配等繁殖产生。此类动物遗传背景明确，具有高度纯合性和稳定性。但由于是高度近交繁殖而成，动物对生长环境要求较高，繁殖力较低。

（2）远交系动物（outbred strains of animals），也称封闭群（closed colony），指在一定群体中进行繁殖，具有杂合性。其生存力、生育力都比近交系强，适合大量繁殖。

（3）杂交一代动物（F1 hybrids），是将两个不同近交品系动物之间进行有计划交配产生的第一代杂交动物。F1 代具有杂交优势，繁殖力强，对外界的适应能力和抗病能力强。并且，这类动物还具有与纯系动物基本相似的遗传匀质性，且表现型一致，基本具有近交系动物的特点，在国际上被广泛应用医学实验研究。

2. 实验动物按微生物控制程度分级

（1）一级，普通动物（conventional animals）。该类动物可在一般自然环境中进行饲养，允许带有寄生虫和细菌，但不允许带有人畜共患病的动物。

（2）二级，清洁级动物（clean-class animals）。这类动物除不能带有人畜共患病的病原体及体外寄生虫、还不能带有动物传染病原体和对实验干扰大的病原体。饲养室必须控制温度、湿度、光照强度和时间。清洁级动物的饲料、饮水及垫料等均须经过消毒处理。

（3）三级，无特定病原体（specific pathogen free，SPF）动物。指体内无特定的微生物和寄生虫的动物，但允许非特定的微生物和寄生虫存在。

（4）四级，无菌动物（germfree animals）。指体内外均无任何微生物和寄生虫的动物。这类动物须在全封闭无菌条件下饲养。

2.1.2 常用实验动物的种属和特性

(1)蟾蜍与蛙：属于两栖纲，无尾目类，变温动物。蟾蜍和蛙的一些基本的生命活动与恒温动物相似，其离体组织器官所需的生存条件比较简单，体外培养存活状态好，因此被广泛用于生理学科科研和教学中。

(2)家兔：属于哺乳纲，啮齿目，兔科。家兔性情温顺，灌胃、取血等操作较方便。兔耳缘静脉部位表浅，易暴露，常用于静脉给药。家兔的减压神经在颈部与迷走神经、交感神经分开而单独成为一束，常用于心血管反射活动、呼吸运动调节、泌尿功能调节的研究。此外，家兔的消化道运动活跃，生理活动典型，可用于消化道运动及平滑肌特性的研究。

(3)小鼠、大鼠：均属于哺乳纲，啮齿目，鼠科。此两种动物均被广泛用于各类科研实验中，如神经科学、药理学、肿瘤学、遗传学、免疫学以及临床疾病的实验研究。

(4)豚鼠　豚鼠属于哺乳纲，啮齿目，豚鼠科，又称荷兰猪。豚鼠耳蜗管发达，听觉灵敏。在生理学上，豚鼠常被用于耳蜗微音器电位及听力的实验研究。

2.1.3 实验动物的选择

生理学实验中，应根据实验目的合理选择动物，实验成败与动物选择是否恰当有密切关系。一般而言，实验动物选择遵循如下原则。

(1)相似性原则。根据实验内容和要求，结合动物解剖生理特点，挑选与人类某些机能、代谢及疾病特点相似的实验动物。

(2)标准化原则。按照实验的特殊要求，选择相应的种属、品种、微生物学背景；保持实验各组别中的动物年龄、体重、性别及健康状况的一致性；实验过程中维持动物饲养环境条件的标准化。

(3)经济化原则。尽量选择价格便宜和饲养方便的实验动物。

2.1.4 动物捉拿和固定方法

在实验过程中，为了手术操作和实验项目记录的方便和顺利开展，必须将动物麻醉并固定在特制的实验台上。固定动物的方法一般多采用仰卧位，它适用于做颈、胸、腹、股等部位的实验。脑和脊髓部位的实验则采用俯卧位。

(1)家兔。对家兔的正确捉持方法为：一手抓住家兔颈背部皮肤，轻轻提起，另一手托住其臀部，使其呈坐位姿势．

(2)小鼠、大鼠。实验者用右手捉住小鼠尾，置于实验台或鼠笼上，并稍向后拉，鼠会本能地向前爬行。用左手拇指和食指抓住小鼠两耳后颈背部皮肤，拉直躯干，并以左手小指和掌部夹住其尾固定在左手上(不熟练者可戴防护手套以防咬伤)。捉持大鼠的方法基本同小鼠。需要注意的是，大鼠在惊恐或激怒时会咬人，捉拿时可戴防护手套，或用厚布盖住鼠身作防护，握住整个身体，并固定头骨，防止被咬伤。

（3）豚鼠。实验者用右手横握豚鼠腹前部，以左手轻托后肢。

（4）蛙。实验者用左手食指和中指控制蛙两前肢，用无名指和小指压住两后肢，拇指轻抵蛙背侧脊柱。

（张先荣）

2.2　实验动物的给药途径

2.2.1　经口给药法

（1）口服法。对实验动物进行口服给药时，可将能溶于水并且在水溶液中较稳定的药物溶于动物饮水中，不溶于水的药物可混于动物饲料内，由动物自行摄入。该方法技术简单，给药时动物接近自然状态，不会引起动物应激反应，适用于多数动物的药物慢性干预实验。但该给药方法存在一定的问题，由于动物本身状态、饮水量和摄食不同，个体间的药物摄入量差异较大，影响药物作用分析的准确性。

（2）灌胃法。对小鼠或大鼠常用的给药方法。实验者用左手固定动物，使动物腹部朝向术者，右手将连接注射器的灌胃针头由口角处插入口腔，用灌胃针头将动物头部稍向后仰，使口腔与食管成一直线，将灌胃针头沿上颚壁轻轻插入食道。插管时应注意动物反应，如插入顺利，动物安静，呼吸正常，可注入药物；如动物剧烈挣扎或插入有阻力，应拔出灌胃针头重插。此外，灌胃时要注意手法轻柔，以防损伤动物口腔和食道黏膜。

2.2.2　注射给药

（1）皮下注射：该注射途径是将药物注射于表皮和真皮下，适合于所有哺乳动物。实验动物的皮下注射一般应由两人操作，熟练者也可一人完成。由助手将动物固定，术者用左手捏起皮肤，形成皮肤帐篷样突起，右手持注射器刺入突起处的皮下，将针头轻轻左右摆动，如摆动容易，表示确已刺入皮下，再轻轻抽吸注射器，确定没有刺入血管后，再将药物注入。

（2）肌肉注射：肌肉注射途径可用于几乎所有水溶性和脂溶性药物。由于肌肉组织内的血管丰富，药物吸收速度快，肌肉注射法特别适用于狗、猫、兔等肌肉发达的动物。小鼠、大鼠和豚鼠因肌肉较少，肌肉注射稍有困难，必要时可选用股部肌肉。肌肉注射一般由两人操作，小动物也可由一人完成。助手固定动物，术者用左手指轻压注射部位，右手持注射器刺入肌肉，回抽针栓，如无回血，表明未刺入血管，再将药物注入。

（3）腹腔注射：腹腔吸收面积大，药物吸收速度快，因此腹腔注射是啮齿类动物常用给药途径之一。腹腔注射部位一般选在下腹部正中线两侧，该部位无重要器官。将动物头部向下、身体稍倒立固定动物，将注射器针头在选定部位刺入皮下，然后使针头与皮肤成20°～30°角缓慢刺入腹腔，回抽针栓，确定针头未刺入小肠、膀胱或血管后，缓慢注入药液。注意：注射器针头尖端不可刺入太深，以防伤及大血管和重要脏器。

（4）静脉注射：将药物直接注入血液，药物作用最快，是急、慢性动物实验最常用的给药方法。采用静脉注射给药时，不同种类的动物由于其解剖结构不同，应根据情况选择合适的静脉血管。

①兔耳缘静脉注射：将家兔置于兔固定箱内，或由助手将家兔固定在实验台上，并特别注意兔头不能随意活动。剪除兔耳外侧缘被毛，用乙醇轻轻擦拭或轻揉耳缘局部，使耳缘静脉充分扩张。用食指、中指夹住耳根，拇指和无名指捏住耳的尖端，右手持注射器由近耳尖处将针刺入血管2～3mm。缓慢推注药物，如感觉推注阻力很大，并且局部肿胀发白，表示针头已滑出血管，应重新穿刺。注意兔耳缘静脉穿刺时应尽可能从远心端开始，以便重复穿刺注射。

②小鼠与大鼠尾静脉注射：小鼠尾部有三根静脉，两侧和背部各一根，两侧的尾静脉更适合于静脉注射。注射时先将小鼠置于鼠固定筒内或倒扣的烧杯中，让尾部露在杯沿外。用乙醇反复擦拭尾部或浸于40～50℃的温水中加温1min，使尾静脉充分扩张。实验者用左手食指和拇指固定尾部注射部位，右手持注射器将针头刺入尾静脉，缓慢注入药物。如推注阻力很大，局部皮肤变白，表示针头未刺入血管或滑脱，应重新穿刺。尾静脉注射可适用于幼年大鼠，操作方法与小鼠相同。成年大鼠尾静脉穿刺困难，不宜采用尾静脉注射。

（张先荣）

2.3 实验动物的麻醉方法

在急、慢性动物实验中，手术前常对动物采用必要的麻醉，以减轻或消除动物的痛苦，并使其处于安静状态，从而保证实验顺利进行。在麻醉时，应根据麻醉药品的作用特点、动物对麻醉药物耐受性的差异和实验内容及要求不同，选择合适的麻醉药品种类、用药剂量及给药途径。

2.3.1 全身麻醉

（1）吸入麻醉：常用的吸入麻醉剂是乙醚，可用于多种动物的麻醉。乙醚麻醉对动物的呼吸、血压无明显影响，麻醉速度快，维持时间短，更适合于时间短的手术和实验，如去大脑僵直、小脑损毁实验等，也可用于凶猛动物的诱导麻醉。麻醉时，一般用倒置烧杯或密闭的玻璃箱等作为容器，将浸润乙醚的棉球置于密闭容器内，然后将待麻醉动物放入。注意：乙醚为无色易挥发的液体，有特殊的刺激性气味，易燃易爆，使用时应远离火源。

（2）注射麻醉：常用乌拉坦、戊巴比妥钠、氯醛糖等，一般采用静脉注射或腹腔注射给药。

2.3.2　局部麻醉

局部麻醉药物通过可逆地阻断神经纤维传导冲动而产生局部麻醉作用，主要有以下两种方式：

（1）表面麻醉：表面麻醉药物可通过滴眼、喷雾或涂布等接触局部黏膜表面，进而透过黏膜作用于黏膜下神经末梢而发挥麻醉效果。该类药物除具有麻醉作用外，还需有较强的穿透力，如的卡因、利多卡因。

（2）浸润麻醉：用注射的方式将麻醉药物送到神经纤维旁。此类麻醉药物只需有局部麻醉作用，不一定要求有强大的穿透力，如普鲁卡因、可卡因、利多卡因。

2.3.3　麻醉效果的观察

动物的麻醉效果直接影响实验的开展和实验结果观察。如果麻醉过浅，动物会因疼痛而挣扎，甚至出现呼吸心跳不规则，影响实验结果；如果麻醉过深，可使动物生理活动的反应性降低，甚至消失，更为严重的是抑制延髓的心血管活动中枢和呼吸中枢，导致动物死亡。因此，在麻醉过程中必须密切观察麻醉程度，判断麻醉效果。

判断麻醉程度的指标有：

（1）呼吸：若动物呼吸加快或不规则，说明麻醉过浅；若呼吸由不规则转变为规则且平稳，说明已达到合适麻醉深度；若动物呼吸变慢，且以腹式呼吸为主，说明麻醉过深动物有生命危险。

（2）反射活动：主要观察角膜反射或睫毛反射。用细棉线或棉球丝轻触动物角膜边缘，若动物的角膜反射灵敏，说明麻醉过浅；若角膜反射迟钝，麻醉程度适宜；角膜反射消失，伴瞳孔散大，则麻醉过深。

（3）肌张力：动物肌张力亢进，一般说明麻醉过浅；动物全身肌肉松弛，说明麻醉合适。

（4）皮肤夹捏反应：麻醉过程中可随时用止血钳或有齿镊以适当力度夹捏后肢皮肤，观察动物反应。若动物反应灵敏，则麻醉过浅；若反应消失，则麻醉程度合适。

观察动物的麻醉效果时，上述四项指标要综合考虑。最佳麻醉深度的标志是：四肢及腹部肌肉松弛、呼吸深慢而平稳、皮肤夹捏反应消失、角膜反射明显迟钝或消失。

2.3.4　麻醉注意事项

（1）麻醉前应正确选用麻醉药品、用药剂量及给药途径。配制适当浓度的药物，以保证注入溶液的体积适中。

（2）进行静脉麻醉时，先将总用药量的三分之一快速注入，使动物迅速渡过兴奋期。余下的药物量则应缓慢注射，并密切观察动物麻醉状态及反应，以便准确控制动物的麻醉深度。

（3）若麻醉较浅，动物出现挣扎或呼吸急促等，需补充麻醉药以维持适当的麻醉效果。一次补充的药量不宜超过原总用药量的五分之一。

（4）麻醉过程中需注意给动物保温，并保持动物的呼吸道通畅。

（5）对于慢性动物实验，实验结束后要监控动物的生理状态。确保动物由麻醉状态苏醒，且能自行翻身或站立为止，才可将动物送回饲养房。

（张先荣）

2.4 常用手术器械

动物生理学实验常用手术器械与医学外科手术器械大致相同，但也有一些专用器械。现仅介绍实验所用的常规手术器械。

（1）手术刀：用来切开皮肤和脏器。手术刀片有圆刃、尖刃和弯刃三种，可根据手术部位和性质选用适当刀片。持刀的方式有 4 种，其中"执弓式"是一种常用的持刀方式。这种持刀方式应用范围广泛而灵活，用于腹部、颈部或股部的皮肤切口。

（2）手术剪和粗剪刀：手术剪尖端有直、弯之分。在生理学实验中，直剪刀主要用于剪皮肤、肌肉等软组织；弯剪刀主要用于剪毛，眼科剪主要用于剪血管和神经等软组织。上述各种手术剪的正确执剪姿势是用拇指与无名指套入剪刀柄的两环，将中指置于无名指环的剪刀柄下，食指压在剪刀轴节处起稳定方向的作用。生理学实验中所用的粗剪刀为普通的家用剪刀。在蛙类的实验中，常用粗剪刀剪蛙的脊柱、骨和皮肤等粗硬组织。

（3）手术镊：常用的手术镊包括有齿镊和无齿镊两种，用于夹住或提起组织，以便剥离、剪断或缝合。一般用有齿镊提起皮肤、皮下组织、筋膜、肌腱等较坚韧的组织，使其不易滑脱。需要注意的是，不能用有齿镊夹持重要脏器，以免损伤器官。无齿镊常用于夹持神经、血管、肠壁等较脆弱组织，而不致使其受损伤。

（4）止血钳：手柄间有齿，可咬合锁住。主要用于夹血管或止血点，以达到止血的目的；也可用于分离组织、牵引缝线，把持或拔缝针等。正确持钳手法和持剪方法相同。打开血管钳的方法是将右手已套入血管钳的拇指与无名指相对按压，继而两指向相反的方向旋开，即可放开血管钳。

（5）骨钳：在打开颅腔和骨髓腔时，可用骨钳咬切骨组织。切勿撕扯，以防撕裂骨膜，损伤脑组织。

（6）颅骨钻：用于开颅时在颅骨表面钻孔。使用时用左手固定颅骨，右手持骨钻。将钻头与骨面垂直，顺时针方向旋转。当钻头到达内骨板时要注意控制钻骨力度，以免穿透骨板而损伤脑组织。

（7）气管插管：在做急性动物实验时，将插管插入气管，以保证呼吸道通畅。

（8）血管插管：包括动脉插管和静脉插管。在做急性实验时进行动脉插管，将插管另一端接压力换能器，可记录动物血压变化。将静脉插管插入静脉后固定，可在实验过程中随时用注射器向静脉血管中注入药物或溶液。

（9）金属探针：用于毁坏蛙类脑和脊髓。

（10）玻璃分针：用于分离神经与血管等组织。

（11）蛙心夹：将夹的前端在蛙心室舒张时夹住心室尖，尾端用细棉线与张力换能器相连。

（12）动脉夹：用于阻断动脉血流。

（13）蛙板：用于固定蛙类的木板。

2.5　哺乳动物实验操作技术

2.5.1　动物固定、剪毛

动物麻醉后需固定于手术台。固定动物的方法和姿势依据具体实验内容而定。常用的固定姿势是仰卧位，适合颈部、胸部、腹部和股部的手术及实验。固定方法是动物仰卧，四根棉绳分别打活结套在动物四肢腕关节和踝关节近端并拉紧，另一端缚于手术台两侧；一根棉绳钩住动物两只上门齿，系缚于手术台前端的铁柱上。还有的固定姿势是俯卧位，适合于颅脑和脊髓实验，用相同的方法固定四肢；头部可以根据实验要求固定于立体定向仪，马蹄形头固定器，或一根棉绳钩住动物上门齿，系缚于手术台前端的铁柱上。侧卧位适用于耳蜗和肾脏的实验。

2.5.2　切开皮肤、皮下组织

根据实验目的和要求确定手术切口的部位和大小。如需要暴露颈总动脉，迷走神经时应选用颈前正中线切口；暴露膈肌时应选在剑突下切口；暴露心脏时应在胸前正中线或左胸部切口；暴露膀胱和输尿管时，应在趾骨联合上方正中切口。切口一般应与血管或器官走向平行，必要时做出标志。进行切口时，用一手拇指和食指向两侧绷紧皮肤使其固定。另一手持刀，使刀刃与欲切开的组织垂直，以适当的力度一次切开皮肤和皮下组织，直至皮下筋膜。组织要逐层切开，并以按皮肤纹理或各组织的纤维方向切开为佳。组织的切开处应选择无重要血管及神经横贯的地方，以免将其损伤。用几把止血钳夹住皮肤切口边缘暴露手术野，以利进一步手术操作。

手术过程中所造成的出血必须及时止住，不仅可以防止继续失血，还可以使手术野清晰。微小血管损伤引起的局部组织渗血，用湿热盐水纱布按压止血。大血管出血，用止血钳将出血点钳住，确认出血点后用丝线结扎。为了避免肌肉组织出血，在分离肌肉时，若切口与肌纤维的方向一致，应钝性分离；若方向不一致，则应采取两端结扎，从中间切断的方法。

创口盖上一块浸以生理盐水的纱布，以防组织干燥。

2.5.3 神经、血管分离技术

神经和血管都是比较娇嫩的组织，在分离过程中要仔细、耐心、轻柔。分离时应掌握先神经，后血管；先细后粗的原则。分离的方向一般要求与神经、血管的走向平行，才能避免损伤组织。在分离较大神经、血管时，应先用止血钳（或眼科镊）将神经或血管周围的结缔组织稍加分离，然后用大小适宜的止血钳插入已被分开的结缔组织破口，沿着神经或血管走向逐渐开大，使神经或血管从周围的结缔组织中游离出来，必要时也可用手术剪将附着在神经或血管上的结缔组织剪去。分离细小的神经和血管时，可用玻璃分针将神经或血管从组织中仔细分离出来。需特别注意保持局部的自然解剖位置。切不可用止血钳或镊子夹持神经和血管，以免受损。分离完毕后，在神经或血管的下方穿以浸透生理盐水的线，备用。

2.5.4 插管技术

1. 气管插管

气管插管的意义在于保持麻醉动物呼吸道通畅，还可以用于收集呼出气体，检测呼吸机能等。气管插管基本方法如下：

(1)于喉部下缘至胸骨上缘之间，沿正中线切开皮肤，钝性分离肌肉组织，暴露、游离出气管，并在气管下穿一较粗的线。

(2)用剪刀于甲状软骨下 1~2cm 处的两软骨环之间，横向切开气管前壁约1/3 的气管直径，再于切口上缘向头侧剪开约0.5cm 长的纵向切口，整个切口呈"T"形。

(3)若气管内有分泌物或血液要用小干棉球拭净。然后一手提起气管下面的缚线，一手将一适当口径的"Y"气管插管由切口向肺插入气管内，用线将气管和插管一起结扎，再缚结于套管的分叉处，加以固定(图 2-1)。

注意事项：

颈部大血管和重要神经均在中线两侧，皮下组织分离一定要顺着肌纤维的方向采用钝性分离。避免损伤大血管和神经。

2. 颈总动脉插管

颈总动脉插管时将一根充满肝素或其他抗凝剂的导管插入颈总动脉，可用于检测动脉血压的变化，也可以用于采集血样。颈动脉插管基本方法如下：

(1)事先准备好插管导管，插入端剪一斜面，另一端连接于装有抗凝溶液（或生理盐水）的血压换能器或输液装置上，让导管内充满溶液，排除气泡。

(2)切开颈部皮肤后，用左手拇指和食指握住夹在切口处皮肤和软组织边缘的止血钳，中指和无名指从外面将皮肤和肌肉轻轻顶起，使颈部气管旁软组织外翻，此时即可见到一侧的血管神经丛。仔细识别该颈总动脉鞘内的颈总动脉。

(3)用玻璃分针仔细分离颈总动脉，游离 2~3cm，穿两根经生理盐水湿润的线于血

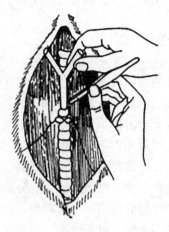

图 2-1　气管插管示意图

管下方备用。

(4)将分离的颈总动脉远心端结扎,近心端用动脉夹夹闭。用眼科剪在靠近结扎处动脉壁成45°剪一"V"字形切口,为管径的1/3~1/2,将动脉插管向心方向插入颈总动脉内,在插入口处将插管与血管结扎在一起,并围绕插管打结、固定。打开动脉夹。(图 2-2)。

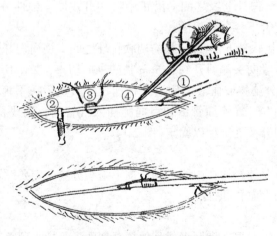

图 2-2　颈总动脉插管示意图

注意事项:

(1)动脉插管需要事先准备好,保证插管部位斜面光滑,避免刺破动脉壁,并且保证插管内肝素水平。

(2)颈总动脉剪口合适,过大则动脉易断,过小不易插入。

3. 胆总管插管

胆总管插管可用于记录胆汁的流量,用于检测胆汁分泌的调节,收集胆汁,胆管插管基本方法如下：

（1）在剑突下正中线切开皮肤约 10cm，显露腹白线，用手术刀或手术剪沿腹白线自剑突向下切开约 10cm。

（2）打开腹腔，将胃向左下方推移，找到胃幽门端，可见与胃幽门连接的十二指肠，将十二指肠向外侧翻转，可见到其壁上隆起的十二指肠大乳头，与圆形隆起相连向右上方行走的一黄绿色较粗的肌性管道，则为胆总管。

（3）用手术弯针在胆总管下方穿线备用。

（4）用眼科剪在十二指肠大乳头上剪口，将插管平行于胆总管向肝胆的方向插入 2~3cm，结扎插管和胆总管，并围绕插管打结、固定。可见黄绿色的胆汁从插管中流出。（图 2-3）。

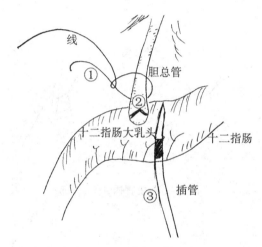

图 2-3　胆总管插管示意图

注意事项：

（1）胆总管壁薄，插管应防止扭曲，避免刺破胆总管或引流不畅。

（2）手术区血管丰富，应避免流血导致手术野不清晰。

4. 输尿管插管

输尿管插管不仅可以观察不同因素对尿量的调控，还可以收集分析尿液成分。输尿管插管基本方法如下：

（1）剪去趾骨联合上方腹部被毛，沿正中线剪开皮肤 4~5cm，显露腹白线，沿腹白线自趾骨联合向上切开约 5cm。

（2）将膀胱牵拉出腹腔，并向下翻转，在膀胱根部两侧辨认输尿管。用玻璃分针分离输尿管，游离 1.5~2cm，在输尿管下穿两根线备用。

（3）用一根线将输尿管膀胱端结扎，提起结扎线，用眼科剪在输尿管近结扎处向肾脏方向成 45°角剪一"V"字形口，为管径的 1/3~1/2，将插管向肾脏方向插入输尿管内 2~3cm，将插管与输尿管结扎在一起，并围绕插管打结、固定。

注意事项：

(1)插管应防止扭曲，避免刺破输尿管或引流不畅。

(2)手术区血管丰富，应避免流血导致手术野不清晰。

5. 膀胱插管

膀胱插管也可以对尿量和尿液成分进行分析，操作相对输尿管插管简单。膀胱插管基本方法如下：

(1)同输尿管插管，牵拉膀胱出腹腔，并向下翻转。

(2)结扎尿道，以防止尿液流出。在两侧输尿管下方、尿道上方穿线，向上翻转膀胱，在膀胱根部结扎尿道。

(3)用两把止血钳夹持膀胱顶部组织并提起，准备好一根固定用的线(图 2-4)，在膀胱顶部血管较少处剪一小口，插入插管 1.5~2cm，将膀胱顶部与插管仪器结扎固定，并围绕插管打结、固定。

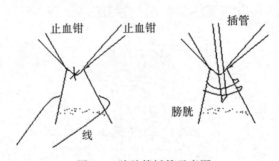

图 2-4　膀胱管插管示意图

注意事项：

(1)膀胱组织有多层，注意不要插入夹层中，插管插入后应立即有尿液流出。

(2)插管不要插入太深，以免组织堵塞导致引流不畅。

2.5.5　取血技术

因实验动物解剖结构和体型大小差异，及所需血量的不同，取血方法不尽相同。

1. 家兔

(1)耳部取血。

可采用耳缘静脉或耳中央动脉取血。首先拔去血管表面皮肤的毛，轻揉耳朵或用酒精涂抹皮肤使血管扩张。用注射器可从耳中央动脉抽取数毫升血。也可用针头刺破耳缘静脉末梢取血。取血后用棉球压迫局部，予以止血。

(2)股动脉取血。

将家兔仰卧位固定。左手以动脉搏动为标志，确定穿刺部位，右手将注射器针头刺入股动脉，如流出血为鲜红色，表示穿刺成功，应迅速抽血，拔出针头，压迫止血。

(3)心脏穿刺取血。

将兔仰卧固定在手术台上，剪去心前区被毛，用 70%酒精消毒皮肤。用左手触摸左侧第 3-4 肋间，选择心跳最明显处作穿刺。装有 7 号针头的注射器刺入心脏后血液一般自动流入注射器，或者边刺入边抽吸。抽血后迅速拔出针头。家兔一次可采取全血量的 1/6~1/5。经 6~7 天后，可以重复进行心脏穿刺术。

2. 大鼠、小鼠

（1）断尾取血。

鼠尾浸泡于 45~50℃ 热水，使鼠尾静脉充分充血后擦干，用剪刀剪去尾尖，血液即可流出，用手轻轻从尾根部向尾尖部挤几下，可以取到数滴血。

（2）眼眶取血。

用左手抓住鼠，拇指和食指尽量将鼠头部皮肤捏紧，使鼠眼球突出。右手取弯钩小镊，在鼠右侧眼球根部将眼球摘去，将鼠倒置头向下，血液从眼眶中流出。取血过程中动物心脏不断在跳动，一般可取出 4%~5% 体重的血液量。

（3）眼球后静脉丛取血。

采用特制的硬玻璃毛细吸管，管长 15cm，直径 1~1.5mm。消毒的吸管用抗凝剂湿润其内壁。取血时，左手抓住鼠，拇指和食指尽量将鼠头部皮肤捏紧，轻轻向下压迫颈部两侧，致静脉回流障碍，从内侧眼角将吸管转向前，并轻压刺入，深 4~5mm 就达到后眼眶静脉丛，血液自然进入吸管内。在得到所需血量后，抽出吸管。

（4）心脏取血。

方法与家兔心脏取血相同，但所用针头可稍短。

2.5.6　动物实验意外处理

动物实验意外是指在实验过程中发生的未预料的事关实验成败的动物紧急情况。常见的动物实验意外如下：

1. 动物麻醉过量

麻醉是动物手术中常见的过程，由于动物的生理状态不同，有时会产生麻醉过量的现象，引起生命中枢麻痹，呼吸缓慢且不规则，甚至呼吸、心跳停止。为了避免麻醉过量，在实际操作中应该注意注射麻醉剂时严格控制注射速度，并密切观察动物呼吸，发现呼吸过度减慢即暂缓或暂停给药。麻醉过量一旦发生，应尽快处理。如动物呼吸极慢而不规则，但心跳仍然存在，应立即施行人工呼吸。以家兔和大白鼠为例，用双手抓握动物腹部，使其呼气，然后迅速放开，使其吸气，频率约为每秒一次。同时，还可以静脉注射尼可刹米（50mg/kg）以兴奋呼吸中枢。如果动物心跳已停止，在人工呼吸的同时，还应做心脏按压。

2. 大出血

在生理实验中，由于操作失误或无法预见的原因，有时会出现大出血。实验动物大出血的预防是非常重要的，手术前一定要熟悉手术部位的解剖结构，以防误伤大血管，分离血管时要仔细、耐心。颈部手术时，钝性分离皮下肌肉和结缔组织。腹部手术时，在腹白线处切开。遇到大出血情况，首先不用慌张，尽快查明出血原因，用棉球吸去血迹，找到出血口点，立即用止血钳钳住出血口的两侧，如出血口不是很大，钳住一段时间后，血液会凝固，此时放开止血钳后不再会出血；如出血口较大，则用止血钳钳住后，再用线将出血口两侧结扎，以防进一步出血。如果是颈动脉插管结扎不紧漏血或插管刺破血管壁出血，应重新结扎或止血后，再重新插管。

3. 窒息

窒息是指动物严重缺氧并伴有二氧化碳蓄积的紧急情况。主要表现为发绀、呼吸极度困难，呼吸频率减慢。大部分实验动物窒息是由于呼吸道阻塞所致，如能及早处理，一般不会造成严重后果；否则实验动物可能因窒息死亡而使实验中止。

慢性动物实验前期手术时不做气管插管，由于麻醉后动物咽部肌肉松弛，常有一定程度的呼吸不畅，严重时可造成窒息。此时，应将动物的舌头向一侧拉出，窒息多可缓解。急性动物实验中，气管插管扭曲堵塞多见于插入端有斜面的插管，其斜面贴于气管壁，造成气道阻塞，这时将气管插管旋转 180°，即可缓解。气管分泌物过多造成气道阻塞时常伴有痰鸣音，血凝块堵塞气管插管可无痰鸣音，可拔出气管插管，并清理插管和气管，再重新插管。

2.5.7　实验动物处死

动物实验结束后，应将动物处死。原则是使动物迅速死亡。

家兔常用处死方法是空气栓塞法，即用注射器向静脉或心脏内注入大量空气，造成广泛空气栓塞，家兔立即痉挛死亡。大鼠和小鼠的常用处死方法是颈椎脱臼法，以左手拇指和食指捏住头部，右手抓住尾部或身体，用力后拉，即可使其颈椎脱臼致死。

动物死亡后应放入指定位置，集中处理。

（童　攒）

第3章 神经-肌肉的信号转导与兴奋反应

实验 1 坐骨神经-腓肠肌标本制备

【实验目的】本实验旨在学习基本的组织分离技术，掌握制备蛙类坐骨神经–腓肠肌标本的制备方法，并获得兴奋性良好的标本。

【实验原理】

两栖类动物的一些基本生命活动规律和生理功能与恒温动物相似，而维持其离体组织正常生理活动所需的培养条件比较简单且易于控制。将离体组织如神经-肌肉标本放在任氏(Ringer's)液中，其兴奋性可在几个小时内维持不变。因此，在生理学实验中常利用蛙的坐骨神经-腓肠肌标本研究神经和肌肉的兴奋性、刺激与肌肉收缩反应的特征及规律等。

【实验对象】

蟾蜍或蛙。

【实验药品与器材】

任氏液，蛙类手术器械(木蛙板、玻璃板、探针、粗剪刀、组织剪、眼科剪、大头针、玻璃分针、滴管、小烧杯、纱布、丝线)，锌铜弓。

【方法与步骤】

(1)破坏脑、脊髓：取蟾蜍一只，用自来水冲洗干净。实验者左手持蟾蜍，使其背部朝上，用拇指按压背部，以食指使头前俯。右手持探针由枕骨大孔处垂直刺入椎管约1mm，然后将探针向前刺入颅腔内，左右搅动探针捣毁脑组织。再将探针退回至枕骨大孔，转向后方刺入椎管(注意将脊柱保持平直)，捻动探针捣毁脊髓。若脑和脊髓破坏完全，蟾蜍下颌呼吸运动消失，四肢完全松软。

(2)剪除躯干上部及内脏：用左手捏住蟾蜍的脊柱，在腰膨大水平上 1cm 处用粗剪刀剪断脊柱。然后将蟾蜍的后肢并拢，以左手握住蟾蜍的后肢，并用拇指抵压脊柱骶部以保持脊柱下段与后肢处于同一水平，这样可使得脊柱横断处上游组织及腹腔脏器自然下垂。沿脊柱两侧将腹壁肌肉及皮肤一并剪至下腹部，再沿耻骨联合处剪去所有内脏，仅保留脊柱和后肢。

(3)剥皮：用左手持镊子捏住脊柱的断端(注意不要触及脊柱两侧的神经)，右手捏住脊柱断端的皮肤边缘，逐步剥去后肢的皮肤。将剥除皮肤的标本置于干净的玻璃板上，滴加少许任氏液备用。将手及使用过的探针、剪刀全部冲洗干净。

（4）分离左右两腿：将标本腹侧向上，左手持镊子夹住脊柱断端的横突，用粗剪刀沿正中线将脊柱及盆骨分为两半（注意，勿伤坐骨神经）。将一半后肢标本置于盛有任氏液的烧杯中备用，将另一半放在玻璃板上进行下一步操作。

（5）游离坐骨神经：将后肢标本脊柱端腹面朝上、并将下肢端扭转至背面朝上，用大头针固定于蛙板上。在近脊柱处穿线结扎神经干，从脊柱根部将坐骨神经干剪断（也可以不结扎、不剪断神经，而保留一小块与神经干相连的脊柱，以便用镊子夹持神经）。用玻璃分针沿脊柱游离坐骨神经至骶部，用剪刀小心剪除骶部的肌肉和结缔组织，暴露深部的坐骨神经。剪断神经走行过程中的小分支及附着的结缔组织。随后在股骨的背侧，用玻璃分针沿股二头肌与半膜肌的肌肉缝纵向分离这两块肌肉，暴露位于两肌肉深部的坐骨神经。将坐骨神经与周边的结缔组织分离，小心剪断坐骨神经的所有分支，一直将神经从脊柱端游离直到腘窝。剪除股骨上附着的肌肉，在股骨中段剪断并去除中段以上其余所有肌肉和骨组织，留取膝关节上方 2~3cm 股骨用于在标本盒中固定标本。

（6）游离腓肠肌：用尖头镊子将跟腱与其下的结缔组织分离，在跟腱处穿细棉线并结扎，在结扎处远端剪断跟腱。用左手提起细棉线，右手持剪刀剪去附着在腓肠肌下方的结缔组织，游离腓肠肌至膝关节处，在膝关节以下将小腿其余部分全剪掉。将制备好的标本浸于任氏液中备用。

【实验项目】

检测标本兴奋性：将标本置于玻璃板上，提起坐骨神经，将锌铜弓浸润任氏液后快速接触坐骨神经，若腓肠肌发生迅速而明显的收缩，表明标本的兴奋性良好。

【注意事项】

（1）损毁蟾蜍脑和脊髓前，先用棉布包裹蟾蜍头部，将其眼后的大腺体挤空，以防腺体分泌液射入操作者眼内。若误入眼内，应迅速用生理盐水冲洗。

（2）制备标本过程中，要经常给标本滴加任氏液，以防止标本因表面干燥而失去正常的兴奋性。

（3）在分离神经和腓肠肌过程中，不可过度牵拉神经和肌肉，且应避免用手或镊子直接接触坐骨神经和腓肠肌。

【思考题】

1. 如何判断蟾蜍的脑和脊髓是否完全损毁？

2. 试述应用锌铜弓检查神经-肌肉标本兴奋性的原理。

【英文专业单词】

坐骨神经-腓肠肌标本（sciatic nerve-gastrocnemius muscle）

兴奋性（excitability）

（张先荣）

实验 2　不同的刺激强度对骨骼肌收缩的影响

【实验目的】

本实验旨在观察电刺激强度变化对骨骼肌收缩张力的影响，理解阈刺激（threshold stimulus）和最大刺激（maximal stimulus）的概念。

【实验原理】

肌肉、神经和腺体组织属于可兴奋组织，具有较高的兴奋性，在受到有效刺激时可产生兴奋。神经组织的兴奋（excitation）表现为动作电位沿神经干的传导，肌肉组织通过兴奋-收缩耦联发生收缩。一般用使细胞发生兴奋所需的最小刺激量来表示组织细胞兴奋性（excitability）的高低。刺激的三要素包括刺激强度、刺激时间和强度-时间变化率。在生理学实验中，通常是将刺激的强度-时间变化率固定，比如用方形电脉冲刺激组织。在一定的刺激时间（波宽）下，刚能引起组织发生兴奋的最小刺激强度称为阈强度（threshold intensity），相当于阈强度的刺激称为阈刺激。能引起组织产生最大兴奋（如肌肉产生最大收缩反应）的最小刺激强度称为最大刺激。

【实验对象】

蟾蜍或蛙。

【实验药品与器材】

Ringer's 溶液、RM6240B 生理信号采集处理系统、蛙类手术器械、标本屏蔽盒、张力换能器、铁支架、双凹夹。

【方法与步骤】

（1）制备蟾蜍（蛙）坐骨神经-腓肠肌标本。

（2）固定标本：将坐骨神经置于标本屏蔽盒的刺激电极上，股骨残端固定于标本屏蔽盒的固定孔内。将腓肠肌跟腱的结扎线与固定于铁支架上的张力换能器相连，并调节结扎线的松紧度（不可过紧或过松）。

（3）连接仪器：将张力换能器的接头插入 RM6240B 生理信号采集处理系统的 CH1 信号输入插孔。将生理信号采集处理系统的刺激输出连接标本屏蔽盒上的刺激电极，如图 3-1 所示。

【实验项目】

在"实验"菜单中选择相应实验模块。在"刺激器"对话框中设置刺激方式为单次，方波正电压，波宽 $0.2 \sim 0.5$ ms，刺激强度从零（或某较低强度）开始以一定"强度增量"逐渐增大。启动刺激，观察肌肉收缩幅度随刺激强度增加的变化。

随着刺激强度增加，将刚能引起腓肠肌收缩的刺激强度称为阈强度，这种刚达到阈强度的刺激称为阈刺激。此后，随着刺激强度的进一步递增，可记录到肌肉收缩曲线的幅度逐步增加。当收缩曲线的幅度不再随刺激强度的增加而升高时，则刚能引起肌肉发生最大收缩反应（收缩曲线的幅度达到最高）的最小刺激强度的刺激，即为最大刺激，如图 3-2 所示。

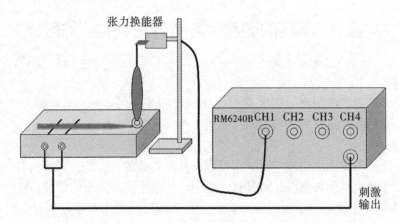

图 3-1　神经-肌肉兴奋收缩装置连接示意图

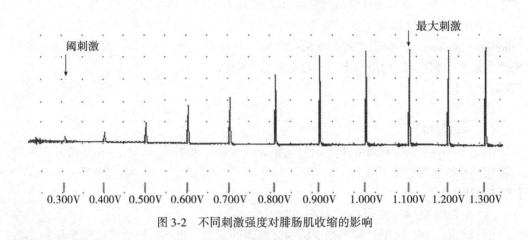

图 3-2　不同刺激强度对腓肠肌收缩的影响

【注意事项】

（1）每完成一轮肌肉收缩实验后，必须间隔一定的时间（0.5~1min）再进行下一轮刺激，以保证肌肉良好的收缩力和兴奋性。

（2）经常用 Ringer's 溶液湿润标本，防止组织标本干燥。

【思考题】

1. 随着电刺激强度的增加，肌肉收缩的幅度有何变化？为什么？

2. 以一定强度电刺激坐骨神经干是如何引起腓肠肌收缩的？

【英文专业单词】

阈刺激（threshold stimulus）　　最大刺激（maximal stimulus）

阈强度（threshold intensity）　　兴奋（excitation）

兴奋性（excitability）

（张先荣）

实验3　不同的刺激频率对骨骼肌收缩的影响

【实验目的】

本实验目的在于观察电刺激频率的变化对骨骼肌收缩形式的影响，记录骨骼肌的几种不同收缩形式：单收缩(single twitch)、不完全强直收缩(incomplete tetanus)、完全强直收缩(complete tetanus)，分析其生理意义。

【实验原理】

骨骼肌的收缩受运动神经纤维支配。神经纤维兴奋后，兴奋沿神经纤维传导，通过神经-骨骼肌接头的化学传递，引起肌细胞产生兴奋(即动作电位)，再经兴奋-收缩耦联使肌纤维中的粗、细肌丝产生相对滑动，肉眼观上表现为肌肉收缩。运动神经元发放冲动的频率会影响骨骼肌的收缩形式和强度。在离体实验中，当运动神经受到一次短促有效的刺激时，可产生一次动作电位，引起其所支配的肌肉出现一次收缩和舒张，这种收缩形式称为单收缩。骨骼肌细胞产生动作电位的时程仅约5ms，而其所诱发产生的骨骼肌收缩过程可达几十或上百毫秒。因此当运动神经受到一定频率的连续刺激时，骨骼肌可以在机械收缩的过程中产生新的兴奋，导致不同兴奋所诱发的收缩过程发生叠加。若刺激频率相对较低，骨骼肌新的收缩过程可与前一次收缩过程的舒张期发生叠加，出现不完全强直收缩。在此基础上继续增加刺激频率，骨骼肌新的收缩过程可与前一次收缩过程的收缩期发生叠加，则肌肉产生完全强直收缩。

【实验对象】

蟾蜍或蛙。

【实验药品与器材】

Ringer's溶液、RM6240B生理信号采集处理系统、蛙类手术器械、标本屏蔽盒、张力换能器、铁支架、双凹夹。

【方法与步骤】

(1)制备坐骨神经-腓肠肌标本。

(2)固定标本：将坐骨神经置于标本屏蔽盒的刺激电极上，股骨残端固定于标本屏蔽盒的固定孔内。将腓肠肌跟腱的结扎线与固定于铁支架上的张力换能器相连，并调节结扎线的松紧度。

(3)连接仪器：将张力换能器的插头插入RM6240B生理信号采集处理系统的CH1信号输入插孔，RM6240B生理信号采集处理系统的刺激输出线连接标本屏蔽盒上的刺激电极。实验装置连接同实验2。

【实验项目】

在"实验项目"菜单中选择相应实验模块。设置刺激参数：固定适当刺激强度，设置波宽0.2~0.5ms。其他参数设置参考如下：

单收缩，频率：1Hz，脉冲数：1；

不完全强直收缩：刺激频率为8~16Hz，脉冲数为5~15；

完全强直收缩：刺激频率为 25~40Hz，脉冲数为 10~25。

不同刺激频率对腓肠肌收缩的影响如图 3-3 所示。

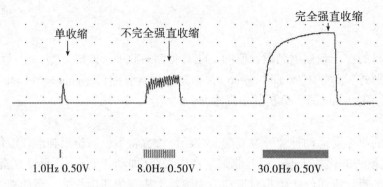

图 3-3　不同刺激频率对腓肠肌收缩的影响

【注意事项】

（1）每完成一轮肌肉收缩实验后，必须间隔一定的时间（0.5~1min）再进行下一轮刺激，以保证肌肉良好的收缩力和兴奋性。

（2）经常用 Ringer's 溶液湿润标本，防止组织标本干燥。

【思考题】

1. 对于同一块肌肉，其单收缩、不完全强直收缩和完全强直收缩的幅度是否相同？为什么？

2. 骨骼肌收缩与心肌收缩的特征有何不同？

【英文专业单词】

单收缩（single twitch）　　　　　不完全强直收缩（incomplete tetanus）

完全强直收缩（complete tetanus）

（张先荣）

实验 4　神经干的动作电位

【实验目的】

学习蛙类坐骨神经干的双相、单相动作电位记录方法，分析复合动作电位的潜伏期、幅值、时程及基本波形。

【实验原理】

以适当强度电刺激兴奋性正常的神经干，在负刺激电极下神经纤维的膜电位产生去极化，当去极化达到阈电位时，即引起动作电位（action potential）的产生。动作电位沿着神经膜传导形成神经冲动。若将一对引导电极置于此神经干表面，则神经冲动先后通过两个电极处，便引导出两个方向相反的电位波形，称为双相动作电位（biphasic action potential)。如果两个引导电极之间的神经纤维完全损伤，神经冲动只通过第一个引导电极，不能传至第二个引导电极，则只能引导出一个方向的电位波形，称为单相动作电位(monophasic action potential)。

神经干由许多不同直径和类型的神经纤维组成，故神经干动作电位与单根神经纤维的动作电位不同。神经干动作电位是由许多神经纤维动作电位叠加而成的综合性电位变化，称为复合动作电位(compound action potential)，其幅度在一定范围内可随刺激强度的变化而变化。

【实验对象】

蟾蜍或蛙。

【实验药品与器材】

Ringer's 溶液、RM6240B 生理信号采集处理系统、蛙类手术器械、标本屏蔽盒。

【方法与步骤】

(1)蛙坐骨神经干标本的制备：方法与制备坐骨神经-腓肠肌标本类似。在靠近脊椎处穿线、结扎坐骨神经干，在线结的上游靠近脊椎处剪断神经。提起结扎线，逐一剪去神经干细小分支，一直将神经干游离至腘窝处。继续向下在腓肠肌两侧肌沟内找到并游离胫神经和腓神经直至足踝。穿线结扎神经，并在结扎线远端剪断神经。将坐骨神经干标本置于 Ringer's 液中备用。

(2)连接实验装置：将刺激电极(S_1 和 S_2，S_2 接刺激的负极)、引导电极(R_1 和 R_1')及地线等接线连好(图 3-4)。提起备用神经干标本的两端扎线，将神经干横搭在标本屏蔽盒的电极上(神经干粗端置于刺激电极处，细端置于记录电极)，盖好屏蔽盒盖。

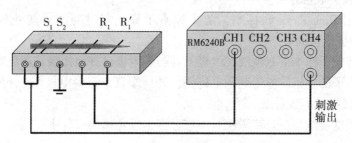

图 3-4 神经干动作电位引导装置连接示意图

(3)实验参数设置：选择相应实验模块，进入实验记录状态。设置刺激器参数，选择"同步触发"正电压刺激方式，模式为单刺激，强度为 0.1~1.0V，波宽为 0.1~0.2ms。

【实验项目】

(1)动作电位幅值与刺激强度之间的关系：在一定范围内增加电刺激强度，神经干复合动作电位的幅度可随刺激强度增加而变化，记录一定刺激波宽时的阈强度和最大刺激强度数值。

(2)双相动作电位：测量最大刺激时双相动作电位的潜伏期、最大峰值和持续时程。

　　(3)单相动作电位：用镊子将两个记录电极之间的神经干夹伤(不要夹断)或用药物(普鲁卡因)局部阻断神经纤维的功能活动。此时再用电刺激坐骨神经干，则双相动作电位的第二相消失，只出现单相动作电位。测量最大刺激时单相动作电位的潜伏期、最大峰值和持续时程。

　　坐骨神经干双相和单相动作电位见图3-5。

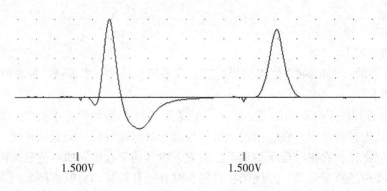

$$1.500V \qquad 1.500V$$

图3-5　坐骨神经干双相和单相动作电位

【注意事项】

　　(1)在分离神经干的过程中切勿损伤神经。夹取神经干标本时须用镊子夹持结扎线头，切不可直接夹取神经干。

　　(2)经常用 Ringer's 湿润标本，防止标本干燥。同时要注意防止标本上过量的 Ringer's 溶液造成电极间短路。

　　(3)应将神经干标本平直地放在电极上并与各电极良好地接触，避免弯曲折叠。

　　(4)将神经干的中枢端置于刺激电极侧，外周端置于记录电极侧。不可将神经组织或两端的结扎线接触屏蔽盒壁。

　　(5)刺激强度要适当，且刺激次数不宜过多，以免损伤神经干。

【思考题】

　　1. 随着刺激强度的逐步增加，神经干复合动作电位的幅度和波形有何变化？为什么？

　　2. 神经干复合动作电位的幅值和图形与单个神经细胞内记录的动作电位是否一样，为什么？

　　3. 神经干双相动作电位的上下波形为何不对称？

　　4. 神经干复合动作电位为什么是双相的？在两个记录电极之间损毁神经后，为什么出现单相动作电位？

　　5. 刺激伪迹是怎么产生的？怎样辨认刺激的伪迹和由刺激引起的动作电位？如何减少或消除刺激伪迹？

【英文专业单词】

动作电位(action potential)　　　　双相动作电位(biphasic action potential)
单相动作电位(monophasic action potential)
复合动作电位(compound action potential)

(张先荣)

实验5　神经干兴奋传导速度的测定

【实验目的】

本实验的目的在于学习神经干动作电位(action potential)传导速度(conduction velocity)的测定和计算方法。

【实验原理】

动作电位在神经干上的传导有一定速度。在不同类型的神经纤维上,动作电位的传导速度不同,神经纤维越粗则传导速度越快。蛙类坐骨神经干以 Aα 类纤维为主,传导速度为 30~40m/s。测定动作电位在神经干上传导的距离(s)与通过这段距离所需时间(t),根据 $v=s/t$ 可计算出动作电位在神经干上的传导速度。在实验过程中,通常采用两个通道同步采集两对引导电极所记录的复合动作电位(compound action potential),以此计算动作电位传导速度。

【实验对象】

蟾蜍或蛙。

【实验药品与器材】

Ringer's 溶液,RM6240B 生理信号采集处理系统、蛙类手术器械、标本屏蔽盒。

【方法与步骤】

(1)蛙坐骨神经干标本的制备(同实验方法4)。

(2)连接实验装置:用镊子夹住神经干标本两端扎线,将标本横搭在屏蔽盒的电极上(将神经干粗端置于刺激电极处,细端置于记录电极)。按图3-6连接实验装置,RM6240B 生理信号采集处理系统的刺激输出端口通过屏蔽导线与标本盒内的刺激电极相连(S_1 和 S_2,S_2 接刺激的负极)。标本屏蔽盒上的 R_1 和 R_1' 及 R_2 和 R_2' 分别是两对记录电极,通过屏蔽导线分别连至计算机的 CH1 及 CH2 信号输入插口。

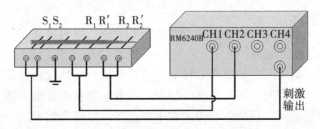

图3-6　神经干动作电位传导速度测定装置连接示意图

（3）实验参数设置：选择相应实验模块，进入实验记录状态。设置刺激器参数，选择"同步触发"正电压刺激方式，模式为单刺激，强度为 0.1 ~ 1.0V，波宽为 0.1 ~ 0.2ms。

【实验项目】

（1）分别测量两个记录电极所记录的神经干复合动作电位的潜伏期（从刺激伪迹到动作电位的起始点之间的时程），用 T_1 和 T_2 表示。两者之间的差值（$T_2 - T_1$）为兴奋沿神经干从 R1 传至 R2 所需的时间（Δt）（如图所示）。在实际测量过程中，由于动作电位的起始点有时难以确定，此时用两复合动作电位第一相电位峰之间的时间差代表 Δt 较为准确。

（2）测量标本屏蔽盒内两对引导电极中起始电极之间的距离（s）。

（3）按公式 $v = s/t$ 计算神经干动作电位（神经兴奋）传导速度，结果如图 3-7 所示。

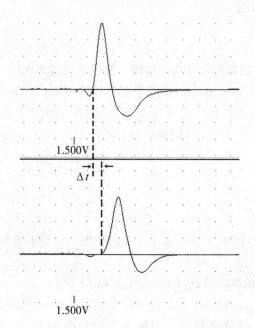

图 3-7　神经干动作电位传导速度的测定

【注意事项】

（1）在分离神经干的过程中切勿损伤神经。提取神经干时须用镊子夹持结扎线头，切不可直接夹神经干。

（2）经常用 Ringer's 溶液湿润标本，防止标本干燥。同时要注意防止标本上过量的 Ringer's 溶液造成电极间短路。

（3）应将神经干标本平直地放在电极上并与各电极良好地接触，避免弯曲折叠。

（4）放置神经干标本时，不可将神经组织或两端的结扎线接触屏蔽盒壁。

（5）刺激强度要适当，且持续刺激次数不宜过多，以免损伤神经干。

【思考题】

　　1. 两对记录电极引导的动作电位在幅度、时程和形状上有无差异？其原因是什么？

　　2. 影响神经纤维传导速度的因素有哪些？

【英文专业单词】

　　动作电位（action potential）

　　传导速度（conduction velocity）

　　复合动作电位（compound action potential）

（张先荣）

第4章 血液生理

实验6 红细胞渗透脆性的测定

【实验目的】

(1)学习红细胞渗透脆性检测方法。

(2)观察红细胞在不同浓度 NaCl 溶液中的形态变化。

【实验原理】

渗透是水分子经半透膜扩散的现象,它由高水分子区域(即低浓度溶液)渗入低水分子区域(即高浓度溶液),直到细胞内外浓度平衡为止。溶液渗透压是指溶液中溶质微粒对水的吸引力。溶液渗透压的大小取决于单位体积溶液中溶质微粒的数目,溶质微粒越多,即溶液浓度越高,对水的吸引力越大,溶液渗透压越高。等渗溶液,指的是渗透量相当于血浆渗透量的溶液,如 0.9%NaCl 溶液。低于血浆渗透量的溶液称为低渗溶液,细胞在低渗溶液中可发生水肿,甚至破裂;高于血浆渗透量的溶液称为高渗液,细胞在高渗溶液可发生脱水而皱缩。

当红细胞置于 0.9%NaCl 的等渗溶液中时,其形态可维持不变;当置于高渗 NaCl 溶液中时红细胞内会失去水分而引起细胞皱缩;当置于低渗 NaCl 溶液中时红细胞会因大量水分进入细胞内而变得膨胀甚至溶血。本实验中将血液加入不同浓度的低渗 NaCl 溶液中,开始出现溶血现象的 NaCl 浓度为红细胞的最大脆性;完全溶血时的浓度为最小脆性。

【实验对象】

家兔。

【实验药品与器材】

(1)实验器材:哺乳动物手术器械、动脉夹、手术台、动脉插管、注射器、试管。

(2)实验试剂:20%乌拉坦、1%NaCl 溶液、灭菌的蒸馏水。

【实验方法】

1. 配制 NaCl 溶液

配制不同浓度的低渗 NaCl 溶液如表 4-1 所示。

Tube No.	1	2	3	4	5	6	7	8	9	10
1%NaCl(ml)	1.80	1.40	1.20	1.10	1.00	0.90	0.80	0.70	0.60	0.50

Tube No.	1	2	3	4	5	6	7	8	9	10
H_2O（ml）	0.20	0.60	0.80	0.90	1.00	1.10	1.20	1.30	1.40	1.50
NaCl （%）	0.90	0.70	0.60	0.55	0.50	0.45	0.40	0.35	0.30	0.25

2. 动物麻醉与固定

耳缘静脉注射乌拉坦(剂量：5ml/kg 体重)，注射时密切观察动物的肌张力、呼吸、角膜反射和痛反射。当麻醉好后将家兔仰卧位固定于手术台上。

3. 动脉插管及血液采集

剪去颈部兔毛，沿正中线做 6~8cm 长切口，钝性分离肌肉，暴露气管。分离一侧的颈总动脉并进行插管，之后进行血液采集。

4. 观察项目

每支试管加入 2 滴血液，然后上下颠倒混匀，静置 1h 后观察结果。

(1)试管内液体分层，下层为浑浊红色，上层为无色透明液体，表明没有发生溶血；

(2)试管内液体分层，下层为浑浊红色，上层为红色透明液体，表明部分红细胞发生破裂，为不完全溶血；

(3)试管内液体不分层，完全为透明红色，表明发生完全溶血。

【注意事项】

(1)小心分离颈总动脉，若有损伤出血，应及时止血；

(2)每支试管所加入的血液量应一致；

(3)血液加入后，应轻轻混匀试管中的液体。

【思考题】

如何分析红细胞的最小脆性和最大脆性？

【英文专业单词】

渗透压(osmotic pressure)　等渗溶液(isoosmotic solution)

（李长勇）

实验 7　血型的鉴定与交叉配血

【实验目的】

(1)学习 ABO 血型鉴定的方法；

(2)了解临床上交叉配血的方法。

【实验原理】

ABO 血型是根据红细胞表面有无特异性抗原(凝集原)A 和 B 来划分的血液类型系统。根据凝集原 A、B 的分布把血液分为 A、B、AB、O 四型。红细胞上只有凝集原 A

的为 A 型血，其血清中有抗 B 凝集素；红细胞上只有凝集原 B 的为 B 型血，其血清中有抗 A 的凝集素；红细胞上 A、B 两种凝集原都有的为 AB 型血，其血清中无抗 A、抗 B 凝集素；红细胞上 A、B 两种凝集原皆无者为 O 型，其血清中抗 A、抗 B 凝集素皆有（表 4-2）。

表 4-2

基因型	细胞表面抗原	血清中抗体	血型
OO	无	Anti-A and anti-B	O
OΛ 或 ΛΛ	Λ	Anti-B	Λ
OB 或 BB	B	Anti-A	B
AB	A 和 B	无	AB

交叉配血试验：受血者血清与供血者红细胞混合，观察受血者血清中是否含有与供血者红细胞反应的抗体。供血者血清与受血者红细胞混合，观察供血者血清中是否含有与受血者红细胞反应的抗体。

【实验对象】

人。

【实验药品与器材】

（1）实验器材：采血针、双凹载玻片。

（2）实验试剂：生理盐水、75%乙醇、A 型和 B 型标准血清。

【实验方法】

将双凹载玻片上分别标记上"A"和"B"，并在相应的小凹中分别加入标准血清 A 和 B，然后分别在小凹中滴一滴血液并混匀，静置观察。

【注意事项】

（1）采血点必须用 75%酒精消毒；

（2）避免 A 型和 B 型标准血清的混合。

【思考题】

血型鉴定的原理是什么？

【英文专业单词】

凝集原（agglutinogen）　血型（blood type）

（李长勇）

实验 8　血液凝固及其影响因素

【实验目的】

分析血液凝固的影响因素。

【实验原理】

血液凝固分为内源性凝血和外源性凝血两种途径，前者是指参与血液凝固的凝血因子全部存在于血浆中，后者是指血液凝固的过程需要组织因子的参与。在本实验中，血液直接从分离的家兔颈总动脉获取，血液未与组织因子接触，所以其凝血过程主要由内源性凝血途径激活所致。

血液凝固是一个复杂的蛋白水解过程，受到多种因素的影响，如温度、接触面的光滑程度以及抗凝剂等物质。

【实验对象】

家兔。

【实验材料】

(1)实验器材：哺乳动物手术器械、动脉夹、家兔手术台、动脉插管、小烧杯。

(2)实验试剂：20%乌拉坦、0.9%NaCl溶液、肝素、草酸钾、液体石蜡。

【实验方法】

1. 动物麻醉与固定

耳缘静脉注射乌拉坦(剂量：5ml/kg体重)，注射时密切观察动物的肌张力、呼吸、角膜反射和痛反射。当麻醉好后将家兔仰卧位固定于手术台上。

2. 动脉插管及血液采集

剪去颈部兔毛，沿正中线做6~8cm长切口，钝性分离肌肉，暴露气管。分离一侧颈总动脉并进行插管。需要放血时，松开动脉夹即可。

3. 观察项目

松开动脉夹，分别取10ml血液加入下列表中各种条件的烧杯中，每隔30s倾斜烧杯一次，观察血液是否凝固，在表4-3中记录各种条件下血液凝固的时间。

表4-3

编号	实验条件	血液凝固时间
1	对照组	
2	在37~40℃水浴	
3	在0℃冰浴	
4	烧杯底部铺上少许棉花	
5	烧杯底部涂上液体石蜡	
6	加少许肝素(8U)	
7	加少许草酸钙(5mg)	
8	用棉签不停搅拌	

【注意事项】

(1)小心分离颈总动脉，如有损伤出血，应及时止血；

（2）每个烧杯中所加入的血液量应一致；

（3）每隔30s倾斜一次，观察是否发生凝固。

【思考题】

实验中各种条件影响血液凝固的具体机制是什么？

【英文专业单词】

血液凝固（coagulation）

（李长勇）

第5章 循环生理

实验9 蛙心起搏点的观察

【实验目的】

(1)学习暴露蛙类心脏的方法，熟悉心脏的结构；

(2)观察改变蛙心局部温度对心脏自动节律性的影响；

(3)用结扎的方法来观察蛙心的起搏点及心脏各部分自动节律性的高低。

【实验原理】

心脏的特殊传导性具有自动节律性，但各部分的自律性高低不同。哺乳类动物以窦房结自律性最高。正常情况下，心脏每次兴奋都从窦房结发出，依次传到心房、心室，相继引起心房、心室收缩，所以窦房结称为哺乳动物心脏的起搏点。两栖类动物心脏的静脉窦的自律性最高，因此静脉窦是起搏点。正常蛙心脏的活动节律服从静脉窦的节律，其活动顺序为：静脉窦、心房、心室。当正常起搏点的下传冲动受阻时，心脏下部节律性较低的部位自动节律性才能表现出来。本实验利用改变心脏局部温度的方法，观察温度对心脏自律性的影响；用斯氏结扎(Straub's ligation)的方法来观察蛙心起搏点和蛙心不同部位自动节律性的高低。

【实验对象】

蟾蜍或蛙。

【实验材料】

(1)实验器材：蛙类手术器械1套、蛙板、大头钉、蛙心夹、离心管、细丝线。

(2)实验药品：任氏液、温水、冰水。

【实验方法】

(1)用探针损毁蟾蜍脑和脊髓，将其仰卧位固定在蛙板上(图5-1)，用镊子提起剑突下端的皮肤，剪开一个小口，然后将剪刀由切口伸入皮下，向左右两侧锁骨外侧方向剪开皮肤，并向头端掀开皮肤。用镊子提起剑突下端腹肌，在腹肌上剪一个小口，将手术剪伸入胸腔内，紧贴胸壁(以免损伤下面的心脏和血管)，沿皮肤切口方向剪开肌肉，再用粗剪刀剪断左右乌喙骨和锁骨，使创口呈一个倒三角形。用眼科镊提起心包膜，并用眼科剪将心包膜剪开，暴露心脏。用蛙心夹于心室舒张期夹住心尖。

(2)观察心脏结构(图5-2)。从心脏的腹面可看到心房、心室及房室沟。心室右上方有一动脉圆锥，是动脉根部的膨大。动脉干向上分成左右两分支。用玻璃分针在心脏

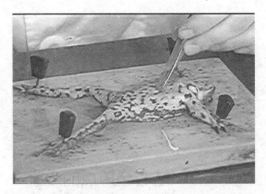

图 5-1　蛙仰卧位固定示意图

背面将心尖翻向头侧，可以看到心房下端有节律搏动的静脉窦。心房与静脉窦之间有一条白色半月形分界线，成为窦房沟。

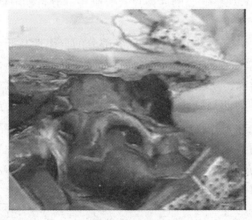

图 5-2　蛙心外观腹侧面照片

【实验项目】

（1）观察正常心搏过程：仔细观察静脉窦、心房和心室的跳动顺序和频率。

（2）改变蛙心局部温度对心脏自律性的影响：用盛有 37℃热水的小离心管和盛有冰水的小离心管分别接触静脉窦或心室以改变它们的局部温度，观察和记录心脏跳动次数的变化。

（3）斯氏第一结扎：将细线沿着窦房沟处进行结扎，此为斯氏第一结扎，以阻断静脉窦和心房之间的冲动传导，观察心脏个部分搏动节律的变化，待心房和心室恢复搏动后（约 15min），分别计数静脉窦、心房和心室的搏动频率。

（4）斯氏第二结扎：待心房和心室及静脉窦搏动恢复正常后，在用细线在房室沟作第二次结扎，此为斯氏第二结扎，以阻断心房和心室之间的传导，观察心房和心室的搏动情况，分别计数静脉窦、心房和心室的搏动频率。

（5）将以上结果填入表 5-1。

表 5-1 　　　　　　　　　　　斯氏结扎记录表

观察项目	搏动频率（次/分钟）			三者频率是否一致
	静脉窦	心房	心室	
正常				
用装有 37℃ 热水的小离心管接触静脉窦				
用装有 37℃ 热水的小离心管接触心室				
用装有冰水的小离心管接触静脉窦				
用装有冰水的小离心管接触心室				
斯氏第一结扎				
斯氏第二结扎				

【注意事项】

（1）经常在蟾蜍心脏上滴加任氏液，使心脏保持湿润。

（2）实验手术操作中，注意保护静脉窦，避免心脏的停搏。

【思考题】

1. 为什么蟾蜍心脏的正常起搏点是静脉窦？

2. 如果在蟾蜍心房和心室的交界处用棉线结扎，心室的跳动会有何变化？

【英文专业单词】

起搏点（pacemaker）

（王媛）

实验 10　期前收缩和代偿间歇

【实验目的】

（1）观察蟾蜍（或蛙）心脏对额外刺激的反应，证明心肌兴奋后兴奋性变化的特点；

（2）学习在体蟾蜍（或蛙）心脏搏动曲线的记录方法。

【实验原理】

心肌细胞每兴奋一次，其兴奋性都会发生一系列周期性的变化。心肌兴奋性的特点是其有效不应期特别长，约相当于心动周期的整个收缩期和舒张早期。在此期间内，任何刺激均不能引起心肌兴奋与收缩。但在舒张期早期以后，给予心室一次阈上刺激，使心室肌在正常窦性兴奋到达前，产生一次提前的兴奋和收缩，称为期前收缩（premature systole）。期前收缩也有自己的有效不应期，若正常的节律性兴奋到达时，正好落在期前收缩的有效不应期内，就不能引起心室的兴奋和收缩。直至下一次正常节律性兴奋到达时，心室才能收缩。心室在期前收缩后出现的一次时间较长的舒张时间，称为代偿间歇（compensatory pause）。

【实验对象】

蟾蜍或蛙。

【实验材料】

（1）实验器材：蛙类手术器械、RM6240 生物信号采集系统、蛙板、蛙心夹、张力换能器、刺激电极、铁支架、双凹夹、小烧杯、滴管。

（2）实验药品：任氏液。

【实验方法】

（1）手术：取蟾蜍一只，用探针破坏脑和脊髓。将其仰卧固定在蛙板上，暴露心脏（参照实验 9）。在心室舒张期用蛙心夹夹住心尖部。

（2）蛙心夹底部穿线与张力换能器相连，使心脏倒立悬挂与胸腔成垂直关系，张力换能器接生物信号采集系统 1 通道。刺激电极插入刺激输出接口，针状电极接触心室表面。

【实验项目】

（1）描记正常心跳曲线，观察心脏收缩期与舒张期相对应的心跳曲线。

（2）选择中等强度的单个阈上刺激，分别在心室收缩期和舒张早期给予刺激，观察能否引起期前收缩。

（3）以同等刺激强度，在心室舒张的中、晚期给予刺激，观察有无期前收缩出现。

（4）若刺激产生了期前收缩，观察是否出现代偿间歇。

【注意事项】

（1）实验过程中，要经常用任氏液保持心脏的湿润。

（2）确保电极在收缩期和舒张期均与心室表面接触。

（3）每刺激一次心室后，要让心脏恢复 2~3 次正常搏动后，再进行下一次刺激。

【思考题】

1. 对记录的曲线加以描述，分析产生期前收缩和代偿间歇的原因。

2. 心肌每发生一次兴奋后，其兴奋性的改变有何特点，其生理意义是什么？

3. 心率过速或过缓时，期前收缩是否会出现代偿间歇？

【英文专业单词】

期前收缩（premature systole）　代偿间歇（compensatory pause）

（王　媛）

实验 11　蛙 心 电 图

【实验目的】

论证机体内容积导体的存在，从而有助于了解由体表引导器官或组织活动的导电规律。

【实验原理】

由于机体任何组织与器官都处于组织液的包围之中，而组织液作为导电性能良好的容积导体，可将组织和器官活动时所产生的生物电变化传至体表。故在体表或容积导体中的远隔部位可记录出某一器官或组织活动的电变化，如心脏活动所产生的生物电变化，可通过引导电极置于体表的不同部位记录下来，即心电图。

【实验对象】

蛙或蟾蜍。

【实验材料】

（1）仪器与器械：RM6240 计算机生物信号采集处理系统、蛙类手术器械、培养皿、大头钉、蛙板。

（2）实验药品：任氏液。

【实验方法与步骤】

1. 手术操作

蛙或蟾蜍毁脑和脊髓后，用大头钉仰卧位固定于蛙板上，暴露心脏（参照实验9）。

2. 连接实验装置

模拟心电图标准导联Ⅱ的连接方式，将接有导线的鳄鱼夹分别夹在固定蛙或蟾蜍右前肢和两后肢的大头钉上，负极接右前肢，正极接左后肢，右后肢则与地线连接，输出导线连接至计算机生物信号采集处理系统（图5-3）。

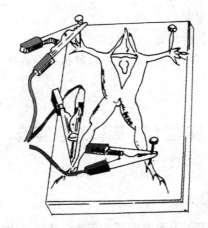

图 5-3　蛙心电图肢体Ⅱ导联连接示意图

3. 实验项目

（1）记录蛙或蟾蜍常规Ⅱ导联时的心电图。

（2）将蛙心用玻璃分针向上翻，使心尖部朝向头部，观察是否能记录到心电图，其波形有何变化。

（3）用蛙心夹夹住心尖部，提起心脏，连同静脉窦一同快速剪下心脏，并将蛙心放入盛有任氏液的培养皿内，观察心电图有何变化。

(4)将培养皿中的心脏重新放回蛙心胸腔原来的位置，观察心电图的变化。

(5)从蛙腿上取下导联线，夹在培养皿边缘并与培养皿内的任氏液相接触，再将心脏置于培养皿中部，心尖朝向正极(图5-4)。观察是否显示心电图波形。

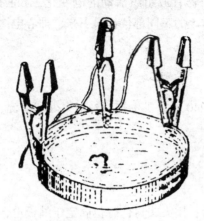

图 5-4　离体蛙心心电图导联连接示图

(6)再将心脏于培养皿内旋转 180°使心尖朝向负极，观察心电图的波形又有何变化。

(7)将心脏从培养皿中去除，观察心电图有何变化。

【注意事项】

(1)用任氏液保持心脏湿润。

(2)剪取心脏时切忌伤及静脉窦。

(3)仪器必须接地良好，以克服干扰。木质蛙板和培养皿应保持绝缘。

（王　媛）

实验 12　离体蛙心灌流

【实验目的】

(1)学习离体蛙心灌流的实验方法；

(2)观察灌流液中几种离子浓度改变对心脏收缩活动的影响，分析其影响机制。

【实验原理】

两栖类动物的离体(in vitro)心脏，用与其内环境相似的任氏液灌流，在一定时间内，仍能维持节律性收缩和舒张。改变任氏液的组成成分，如改变 Na^+、K^+、Ca^{2+} 的浓度及酸、碱度等，心脏跳动的频率和幅度就会发生相应的改变。

【实验对象】

蟾蜍或蛙。

【实验材料】

(1)装置和器材：蛙类手术器械、RM6240 生物信号采集处理系统、蛙板、蛙心夹、蛙心插管、铁支架、双凹夹、蛙心插管固定夹、棉线、张力换能器。

（2）试剂和药品：任氏液、0.65% NaCl、1% KCl、2% CaCl₂、3% 乳酸、2.5% NaHCO₃、1：10000 肾上腺素、1：100000 乙酰胆碱。

【实验方法】

（1）破坏蟾蜍脑和脊髓，暴露心脏。

（2）在主动脉左侧分支下穿两根线，右侧分支下穿一根线，动脉主干下穿一根线备用。先结扎动脉干右侧分支，再用玻璃针将心脏翻至背面，在静脉窦以外结扎前后腔静脉（注意勿扎住静脉窦）。将心脏翻至腹面结扎动脉干左侧分支远端，然后用眼科剪刀在左侧分支近心端剪一斜口。取一蛙心插管，注入适量任氏液于管内，用右手拇指堵住插管外口，食指和无名指夹持蛙心插管，用左手提起动脉干左侧分支远端结扎线，将蛙心插管的尖端自斜口插入动脉腔内，插至动脉圆锥时略向后退，在心室收缩时，沿心室后壁方向向下插入心室。（图 5-5 和图 5-6）插管进入心室后，管内液面会随着心室跳动而上下波动。最后用近心端备用线结扎并固定蛙心插管和动脉管壁，并将结扎线固定于插管侧壁的小突起上。提起插管，在结扎线远心端分别剪断动脉干左、右侧分支和前、后腔静脉，将心脏离体。随即用任氏液反复换洗插管内液体至完全澄清。用双凹夹将蛙心插管固定于铁支架上备用。在心室舒张时，用蛙心夹夹住心尖约 1mm，将蛙心夹上的棉线连接到张力换能器上，再将张力换能器连接到计算机的相应接口。启动计算机并开启生物信号采集处理系统。

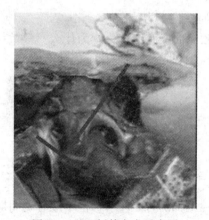

图 5-5 蛙心插管方向示意图

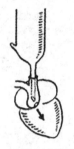

图 5-6 蛙心插管模式图

【观察项目】

（1）描记正常心脏收缩曲线：曲线幅度代表心室收缩的强弱，单位时间内的曲线个数代表心跳频率。曲线向上移动表示心室收缩，其顶点水平代表心室收缩所达到的最大程度；曲线向下移动表示心室舒张，其最低点即基线水平代表心室舒张的最大程度。

（2）吸出插管内全部任氏液，换入 0.65%NaCl，观察心搏曲线变化，待效应出现后，用新鲜任氏液反复换洗直至心搏曲线恢复正常。

（3）加入 1~2 滴 2%CaCl₂ 于任氏液中，观察心搏曲线的变化，待效应出现后，用新鲜任氏液反复换洗至曲线恢复正常。

(4)加入 1~2 滴 1%KCl 于任氏液中，观察心搏曲线的变化，待效应刚出现时，立即用新鲜任氏液反复换洗直至心搏曲线恢复正常。

(5)加入 1~2 滴 1：10 000 肾上腺素，观察心搏曲线的变化，待效应出现后，用新鲜任氏液反复换洗直至心搏曲线恢复正常。

(6)加入 1 滴 1：100 000 的乙酰胆碱，观察心搏曲线的变化，待效应刚出现时，立即用新鲜任氏液反复换洗直至心搏曲线恢复正常。

(7)加入 1 滴 3% 乳酸，观察心搏曲线的变化，待效应出现后，加入 1 滴 2.5% NaHCO$_3$，再观察心搏曲线的变化，至心搏曲线基本恢复时，再用新鲜任氏液反复换洗直至心搏曲线恢复正常。

【注意事项】

(1)实验过程中，要经常用任氏液保持心脏的湿润。

(2)当每种化学药物(尤其是抑制心脏活动的药物)作用已明显时，应立即换洗，以免心肌受损。反复用任氏液换洗数次，待心跳恢复正常后再进行下一步实验。

(3)做每项实验时均应保持插管内的液面在相同高度。

(4)不同药物之间不能混用滴管，以免影响实验结果。

【思考题】

1. 用 0.65% NaCl 替换任氏液后，心脏收缩曲线有何变化？为什么？

2. 滴加 1%KCl 后，心脏收缩曲线有何变化？为什么？

3. 滴加 3%CaCl$_2$后，心脏收缩曲线有何变化？为什么？

4. 滴加 1：10 000 肾上腺素后，心脏收缩曲线有何变化？为什么？

5. 滴加 1：100 000 乙酰胆碱后，心脏收缩曲线有何变化？为什么？

(王　媛)

实验 13 人体心音听诊

【实验思路与目的】

本实验以人体为研究对象，用听诊器在胸部的各瓣膜听诊区听取心动周期中心脏搏动的声音。目的是学习人体心音听诊的方法，识别第一心音与第二心音，了解正常心音特点及其产生原理。

【实验原理】

心动周期(cardiac cycle)中，心肌收缩，瓣膜启闭，血液流速改变对心血管壁的作用以及形成的涡流等因素引起的机械振动，可通过周围组织传递至胸壁。用听诊器可以在胸部听到这些振动所产生的声音，称为心音(cardiac sound)。正常心脏在一次搏动中可产生 4 个心音。多数情况下只能听到第一心音和第二心音。①第一心音：音调较低、持续时间较长，是由心室射血时涡流的血液撞击扩张的大血管壁引起的动脉壁振动和房室瓣突然关闭引起的室壁振动所产生的。由于房室瓣的关闭与心室收缩开始几乎同时发生，因此第一心音标志心室收缩的开始，其响度和性质变化常可反映心室肌收缩强、弱和房室瓣膜的机能状态。②第二心音：音调较高而持续时间较短，其产生主要由半月瓣关闭产生振动造成的。由于半月瓣关闭与心室舒张开始几乎同时发生，因此第二心音标志心室舒张的开始，其响度常可反映动脉压的高低。结合触诊心尖搏动（cardiac impulse）或颈动脉搏动（carotid impulse）有助于心音的听诊（auscultation）。临床常用的心音听诊区如图 5-7 所示。

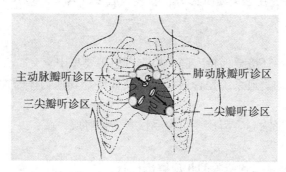

图 5-7　心音听诊部位示意图

【实验对象】

人（志愿者）。

【实验器材】

听诊器、秒表。

【实验方法与步骤】

1. 戴好听诊器

（1）听诊器由耳件、胸件和橡皮导管组成。

（2）佩戴使用听诊器时，耳件方向应与外耳道方向一致，以右手拇指、食指和中指轻持听诊器胸件。

2. 确定听诊部位

受试者多采取仰卧位或坐位，解开上衣，面向亮处，检查者站在床的右侧或坐在受试者对面。注意观察或用手触诊受试者心尖搏动的位置和范围。

心脏瓣膜听诊区为四个瓣膜五个区，如图 5-7 所示。①二尖瓣听诊区：左锁骨中线稍内侧第五肋间（心尖部）；②三尖瓣听诊区：胸骨右缘第四肋间或剑突下；③主动脉瓣听诊区：胸骨右缘第二肋间；④主动脉瓣第二听诊区：胸骨左缘第三肋间；⑤肺动脉瓣听诊区：胸骨左缘第二肋间。

3. 熟悉听诊顺序

听诊顺序一般按瓣膜听诊区循逆"8"字笔画方向依次听诊，即从二尖瓣听诊区→主动脉瓣听诊区→肺动脉瓣听诊区→三尖瓣听诊区。

【实验项目】

1. 听心音

（1）根据心音的响度和音调、持续时间、时间间隔等，仔细区分第一心音和第二心音。

(2)若难以分辨两个心音,听诊时可用手指触摸心尖搏动或颈动脉搏动,心音与心尖搏动或颈动脉搏动在时间上有一定关系,利用这种关系,有助心音的辨别。

(3)比较各瓣膜听诊区两心音的声音强弱(intensity of cardiac sound)。

(4)判断心音的节律(cardiac rhythm)是否整齐。

2. 数心率(Heart rate,HR)

将听诊器的胸件放在二尖瓣听诊区,看表数心率。若节律整齐,可只数 15s 的心跳次数,其 4 倍即为心率。

【注意事项】

(1)心音听诊时,环境要保持安静,检查者思想要集中。

(2)检查听诊器的管道系统是否通畅。硅胶管勿与其他物体摩擦,以免发生摩擦音影响听诊。

(3)如果呼吸音影响心音听诊,可令受试者暂停呼吸。

【思考与评价】

1. 心音听诊区是否在各瓣膜的相应解剖位置?

2. 怎样区别第一心音和第二心音?

3. 评价:心脏的某些异常活动可以产生杂音或其他异常的心音。因此听取心音对于心脏疾病的诊断具有重要意义。

【英文专业单词】

心音(cardiac sound)　　　听诊(auscultation)

心率(heart rate,HR)　　　心律(cardiac rhythm)

(严晓红)

实验 14　人体动脉血压测量

【实验目的】

本实验通过临床常用的无创、简便的间接测量血压的方法测定人体上臂肱动脉的血压,用来代表该个体的动脉血压。目的是学习间接测定人体动脉血压的原理和方法,测量人体肱动脉的收缩压与舒张压。

【实验原理】

用血压计进行人体动脉血压(arterial blood pressure)间接测量最常用的方法是袖带法,即用血压计(sphygmomanometer)的袖带(cuff)在动脉外施加压力,根据血管音(Korotkoff sound)的变化来测量(measurement)血压的数值,又称 Korotkoff(克罗特科夫)听诊法。通常血液在血管内流动时并没有声音,如果血流经过狭窄处形成涡流,则发出声音。用袖带(图 5-8)在上臂给肱动脉(brachial artery)加压,当外加压力超过动脉的收缩压时,完全阻断了肱动脉内的血流,此时用听诊器在肱动脉处听不到声音,也触不到桡动脉(radial artery)的搏动。当袖带内压力稍低于肱动脉收缩压的瞬间,血液通过受压而变窄的肱动脉形成涡流而发出声音，此时血压计的压力读数即为收缩压（systolic pressure）。同时若触诊桡动脉，也可触到桡动脉脉搏。当袖带内压力越接近于舒张压时，通过的血量越多，并且血流持续时间越长，听到的声音越来越强而清晰；当袖带内的压力等于或稍低于舒张压瞬间，血管内的血流由断续变为连续，血管处于通畅状态，因不能形成湍流，血管音突然由强变弱或消失，脉搏随之恢复正常，此时袖带内的压力即为舒张压（diastolic pressure）。

【实验对象】

人。

【实验器材】

血压计、听诊器、手表。

【实验方法与步骤】

1. 了解血压计的结构

目前血压计有三种，即水银柱式、表头式和电子血压计。血压计主要由检压计、袖带和橡皮球（电子血压计除外）组成。其中水银检压计是一个有 0～260mm 刻度的玻璃管，上端与大气相通，下端与水银槽相通；表头式检压计是一个带有指针和刻度的表盘，压力可推动指针在表盘上旋转到某一刻度。袖带是一个外包布套的长方形橡皮囊，借橡皮管分别与检压计的水银槽及橡皮球相通。橡皮球是一个带有螺旋阀的球形橡皮囊，供充气和放气用。电子血压计只有电子表盘和袖带两部分组成，可由电子表盘上的开关控制自动充气、放气和显示血压值。

2. 间接测量动脉血压的方法

测量时，被测者一般取坐位或平卧位，上臂的中点与心脏保持同一水平位。测量者通过扣诊触及动脉搏动以定位肱动脉，将血压计袖带以适当的松紧度缠绕在被测者上臂，袖带下缘位于肘弯横纹上方 2～3cm 处。听诊器膜型胸件置于肘窝部，肱二头肌内侧的肱动脉搏动处。然后向袖带内的气囊充气加压，当所加压力高于收缩压时，该处的肱动脉血流被完全阻断，肱动脉搏动消失，此时在听诊器上听不到任何声音，继续充气使汞柱再升高 20～30mmHg，随后以 2～3mmHg/s 的速度缓慢放气，当袖带内的压力稍低于收缩压的瞬间，血流突入被压迫阻塞的血管段，形成湍流撞击血管壁，此时听到的第一次声响（Korotkoff sound）的血压计汞柱读数即为收缩压。当袖带内压力降到等于或稍低于舒张压时，血流完全恢复畅通，听诊音消失，此时的汞柱读数为舒张压。

3. 血压记录的书写方式

常以收缩压/舒张压 mmHg 表示。

4. 测量动脉血压前的准备

（1）受试者静坐 5～10min，脱掉被测上肢（常为右上肢）衣袖，采取仰卧位或坐位，肘部应与心脏处于同一水平，上臂伸直并轻度外展（图 5-8）。

（2）检查者松开血压计橡皮球螺旋阀，将袖带展平，排尽空气，再旋紧螺旋阀。

（3）将袖带气囊部分对准肱动脉，紧贴皮肤缠于上臂，袖带下缘应距肘关节上 2～3cm 处，松紧应适宜。

（4）检查者戴好听诊器，先在肘窝处触到肱动脉搏动，再将听诊器的胸件置于肘窝

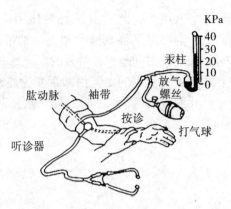

图 5-8 人体动脉血压测量方法示意图

处肱动脉上，轻压听诊器胸件与皮肤紧密接触。

【实验项目】

(1)测量收缩压：挤压气球，向袖带内充气加压，边充气边听诊，将水银柱升高至约 180mmHg，或待肱动脉搏动消失后，继续充气将水银柱升高 20~30mmHg，松开气球螺旋阀，缓慢放气，两眼平视汞柱，仔细听诊，听到第一声响时的汞柱液面所指示的刻度数值即为收缩压。

(2)测量舒张压：继续缓慢放气，随汞柱下降，声音逐渐加强，继而出现吹风样杂音，然后声音突然变小而低沉，最后声音消失，声音消失时汞柱所指示的刻度数值即为舒张压。

【注意事项】

(1)室内必须保持安静，以利听诊。

(2)袖带应缚于肘窝以上至少 2cm，将胸件置于肱动脉搏动处，切不可将其插入袖带下测量。袖带的缠绕不宜过松或过紧，以可插入一指头为宜。

(3)动脉血压通常可连续测 2 次，但必须间隔 3~5min。重复测定前，必须使袖带内的力降到零位。一般取两次较为接近的数值为准。

(4)测压部位的位置应与心脏同高，上臂位置应与右心房同高。

(5)如血压超出正常范围，应让受试者休息 10min 后再测。受试者休息期间，可将袖带解下。

(6)左、右肱动脉可有 0.7~1.3kPa(5~10mmHg)的压力差，测量时固定在一侧上臂不得随意更换。

(7)注意正确使用血压计，开始充气时打开水银柱根部的开关，使用完毕后应将袖带内气体驱尽，卷好，放置盒内。将检压计向右略倾斜，使管内水银退回储槽内，再关上开关，以免水银泄漏。

【思考与评价】

1. 何谓收缩压和舒张压？其正常值是多少？

2. 说明收缩压和舒张压的测定原理。

3. 测血压时，听诊器的胸件为什么不能插入袖带下？

4. 在短时间内为什么不能反复多次测量动脉血压？

5. 评价：用 Korotkoff 音听诊法测得的动脉收缩压和舒张压与直接测量法相比，相差不足 10%。

【英文专业单词】

动脉血压(arterial blood pressure)　　　　肱动脉(brachial artery)

收缩压(systolic pressure)　　　　　　　　舒张压(diastolic pressure)

（严晓红）

实验 15　心血管活动的神经体液调节

【实验目的】

(1)学习记录哺乳动物动脉血压的直接测定方法。

(2)观察神经-体液因素对心血管活动的调节。

【实验原理】

生理情况下，哺乳动物的血压处于相对稳定状态，这种相对稳定是通过神经和体液因素的调节而实现的。在神经调节中以颈动脉窦-主动脉弓的压力感受性反射尤为重要，该反射既可在血压升高时降压，又可在血压降低时升压。反射的传入神经为主动脉神经和窦神经。家兔的主动脉神经为一条独立的神经，也称减压神经，易于分离和观察其作用。反射的传出神经为心交感神经、心迷走神经和交感缩血管神经纤维。心交感神经兴奋，其末梢释放去甲肾上腺素，去甲肾上腺素与心肌细胞膜上的 β 受体结合，引起心脏正性的变时变力变传导作用；心迷走神经兴奋，其末梢释放乙酰胆碱，乙酰胆碱与心肌细胞膜上的 M 受体结合，引起心脏负性的变时变力变传导作用；交感缩血管纤维兴奋时释放去甲肾上腺素，后者与血管平滑肌细胞的 α-受体结合，使外周阻力增加。

【实验对象】

家兔。

【药品与器材】

(1)药品：20%氨基甲酸乙酯溶液、肝素、1∶10 000 去甲肾上腺素、1∶100 000 乙酰胆碱、阿托品、生理盐水。

(2)器材：RM6240 生理信号采集处理系统、哺乳类动物手术器械一套、气管插管、血压换能器、动脉插管、动脉夹、刺激电极、注射器及针头、玻璃分针、纱布、铁支架、棉绳。

【方法与步骤】

(1)麻醉和固定：用 20%氨基甲酸乙酯溶液，按 5ml/kg 体重剂量从耳缘静脉注入体内，待动物麻醉后，背位固定于兔台上。

(2)准备动脉插管：通过三通管将血压换能器与动脉插管中注入 0.5%肝素。消除气泡。

(3)分离颈部神经和血管：剪去颈部兔毛，于颈部正中切开 6~8cm 皮肤和皮下组织。钝性分离肌肉，暴露气管。左手握住夹在切口处皮肤和软组织边缘的止血钳，以食指作后衬，使颈部气管旁软组织外翻，此时即可见到一侧的血管神经丛。仔细识别该颈总动脉鞘内的结构：颈总动脉、迷走神经、交感神经和减压神经。迷走神经最粗，减压神经最细(图 5-9)。

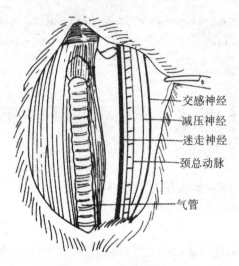

图 5-9　兔颈部神经、血管解剖位置示意图

(4)用玻璃分针仔细分离迷走神经和减压神经，游离 2cm 左右，穿一根经生理盐水湿润的线于神经下方备用。用玻璃分针分离颈总动脉，穿两根经生理盐水湿润的线于血管下方备用。

(5)动脉插管：将分离的颈总动脉远心端结扎，近心端用动脉夹夹闭。用眼科剪在靠近结扎处动脉壁剪一"V"字形切口，将动脉插管向心方向插入颈总动脉内，扎紧固定。打开动脉夹。

(6)血压换能器接入通道 1。

【实验项目】

(1)记录一段时间的正常血压曲线(图 5-10)。

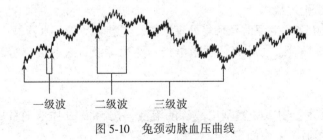

一级波　　二级波　　三级波

图 5-10　兔颈动脉血压曲线

曲线包括：①一级波(心搏波)，是指由心室的舒缩活动引起的血压波动。心缩时

上升，心舒时下降，其频率与心率一致。②二级波（呼吸波），是指由呼吸时肺的张缩所引起的血压波动。吸气时，血压先降低然后升高；呼气时，血压先升高然后降低。③三级波（不常见到），产生原因未完全清楚，可能是由于血管运动中枢紧张性的周期性变化的结果。

（2）夹闭颈总动脉：动脉夹夹闭另一侧颈总动脉 5~10s，然后松开动脉夹。记录夹闭和放松颈总动脉前后的动脉血压及心率变化。

（3）牵拉颈总动脉：持插管侧颈总动脉远心端结扎线，向心脏方向拉紧，有节奏地往复牵拉 5~10s。记录动脉血压及心率变化。

（4）耳缘静脉注射 1∶10 000 去甲肾上腺素 0.2~0.3 ml，记录注射前后的动脉血压及心率的变化。

（5）耳缘静脉注射 1∶100 000 乙酰胆碱 0.2~0.3 ml，记录注射前后的动脉血压及心率的变化。

（6）耳缘静脉注射阿托品 0.5 ml，1~2 min 后再注射 1∶100 000 乙酰胆碱 0.2~0.3 ml，记录注射前后的动脉血压及心率的变化。

（7）电刺激减压神经：使用刺激保护电极以中等频率（20 Hz）和强度（3~5 V）刺激减压神经，记录刺激前后的动脉血压及心率的变化。在减压神经中部做双重结扎，结扎线中间剪断神经，以同样刺激参数分别刺激其中枢端和外周端，记录刺激前后的动脉血压及心率的变化。

（8）电刺激迷走神经：结扎左侧迷走神经，靠近中枢端剪断，使用刺激保护电极以中等频率（20Hz）和强度（5~10V）刺激（10s）迷走神经外周端，记录刺激前后的动脉血压及心率的变化。

（9）改变体位：迅速抬起家兔的头部，维持 2~5s，观察和记录改变体位前后的动脉血压的变化。将动物放平后，迅速抬起家兔的下肢，维持 2~5s，记录改变体位前后的动脉血压及心率的变化。

【注意事项】

（1）麻醉要适量，过浅则家兔挣扎；过深则反射不灵敏且容易引起家兔死亡。

（2）动脉插管与动脉方向保持一致，既可使血液压力顺利传送到血压换能器，又可防止插管刺破血管。

（3）观察完每一项实验后，必须等到血压基本恢复正常，再进行下一个实验项目。

（4）注意保护耳缘静脉。每次注射药物后立即再注射 0.5ml 生理盐水，以防止药液残留在针头及局部静脉中而影响下一种药物的效应。

（5）分离神经要用玻璃分针，不能牵拉神经使神经受损。经常用生理盐水湿润神经，以免影响刺激效果。

【思考与评价】

试分析各实验因素引起动脉血压变化的机制。

【英文专业单词】

心率（heart rate） 神经体液调节（neural and humoral regulation）

（童 攒）

实验 16　减压神经放电

【实验目的】

(1)了解引导神经放电的电生理实验方法。

(2)观察家兔减压神经放电波形的特点。

【实验原理】

多数哺乳动物主动脉弓压力感受器的传入神经在颈部并入迷走神经，进入延髓。兔的主动脉弓压力感受器的传入神经纤维自成一束，在颈部与迷走神经、交感神经并行，称为减压神经。减压神经在动脉血压的调控中发挥重要的作用，当动脉血压升高时，主动脉弓压力感受器的传入冲动增多，经减压神经传入中枢，调节血压下降；反之，当动脉血压降低时，主动脉弓压力感受器发放冲动减少，经减压神经传入中枢，调节血压升高。因此，在一个心动周期内，随着动脉血压的波动，减压神经的传入冲动也发生周期性的变化。

【实验对象】

家兔。

【药品与器材】

(1)药品：20%氨基甲酸乙酯溶液、肝素、1∶10 000 去甲肾上腺素、1∶100 000 乙酰胆碱、生理盐水、液体石蜡。

(2)器材：RM6240 生理信号采集处理系统、哺乳类动物手术器械一套、音箱、血压换能器、气管插管、动脉插管、动脉夹、记录电极、注射器及针头、玻璃分针、纱布、铁支架、棉绳。

【方法与步骤】

(1)麻醉和固定：用 20%氨基甲酸乙酯溶液，按 5ml/kg 体重剂量从耳缘静脉注入体内，待动物麻醉后，背位固定于兔台上。

(2)手术：剪去颈部兔毛，于颈部正中切开皮肤。分离气管，作气管插管术。左手握住夹在切口处皮肤和软组织边缘的止血钳，以食指作后衬，使颈部气管旁软组织外翻，此时即可见到一侧的血管神经丛。用玻璃分针仔细分离同侧的减压神经(它在与迷走神经、交感神经三者中为最细)。游离 2cm 左右，穿一根经生理盐水湿润的线于神经下方备用。

(3)动脉插管：分离一侧颈总动脉进行动脉插管术，描记血压(方法参照心血管活动的神经体液调节)。通道 2 记录动脉血压。

(4)引导减压神经放电：用钩状电极将减压神经勾起，并使电极悬空，不要接触周围组织；把电极固定在支架上，然后用止血钳将颈部皮肤提起拉开，做一皮兜，滴入 38℃的液体石蜡，以保温和保湿。记录电极输入通道 1。

【实验项目】

　　(1)记录一段时间的正常曲线,观察减压神经放电的群集放电的节律、波形和幅度(图 5-11),分析减压神经放电与血压波动的关系。

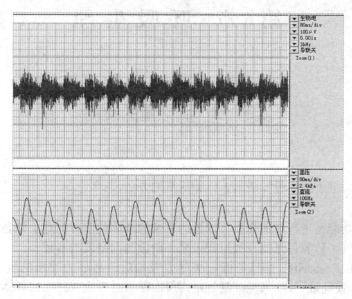

图 5-11　兔的减压神经群集放电和血压

　　(2)生物信号采集处理系统连接音箱,监听减压神经放电的声音,类似火车开动的声音。

　　(3)向耳缘静脉注入 1∶100 000 乙酰胆碱 0.2~0.3 ml,观察血压与减压神经群集放电频率的变化以及二者的关系。

　　(4)待血压恢复稳定后,由耳缘静脉注入 1∶10 000 去甲肾上腺素 0.2~0.3 ml,观察血压与减压神经群集放电频率的变化以及二者的关系。

【注意事项】

　　(1)小心分离减压神经,分离后立即加入温的液体石蜡,勿伤及血管,若电压降低,可将引导电极向近心端移动。

　　(2)麻醉动物不宜过浅,引导电极不接触周围组织,尽量排除干扰。

【思考与评价】

　　1. 阐述减压神经放电与动脉血压的关系。

　　2. 阐述乙酰胆碱和去甲肾上腺素影响减压神经发电的机制。

【英文专业单词】

减压神经(depressor nerve)　　　压力感受性反射(baroreceptor reflex)

(童　攒)

第6章 呼吸生理

实验17 肺活量的检测

【实验目的】

学习与掌握电子肺活量计测量人体肺活量的方法。

【实验原理】

肺的主要功能是进行气体交换，以维持正常的新陈代谢。为此，肺必须与外界大气不断地进行通气。肺容量是指呼吸过程中某一阶段肺内空气的容积。

肺活量(vital capacity, VC)是指一次尽力吸气后，再尽力呼出的气体总量。肺活量=潮气量+补吸气量+补呼气量。潮气量指每次呼吸时吸入或呼出的气体量。补吸气量又称吸气储备量，指平静吸气末，再尽力吸气所能吸入的气体量。补呼气量又称呼气储备量，指平静呼气末，再尽力呼气所能呼出的气体量。肺活量是一次呼吸的最大通气量，在一定意义上可反映呼吸机能的潜在能力。成年男子肺活量约为3 500ml，女子约为2 500ml。

肺通气量则为单位时间内通过肺的气体流通量。常用肺活量计用来测量肺通气量。

【实验对象】

人。

【药品与器材】

电子肺活量计、一次性吹嘴。

【方法与步骤】

(1)接通电源并开机调零。

(2)受测者尽力深吸气直到在不能吸气时，将嘴对准吹嘴做一次尽力深呼气，直到再不能呼气为止。此时显示器上显示的值即为受试者的肺活量值。

(3)连续测试三次，记录并显示最大值。

【实验项目】

在下表中记录平静状态下的肺活量。

肺活量测定表

	第1次	第2次	第3次
肺活量(毫升)			

【注意事项】

(1)检测时应注意防止从鼻孔或嘴角漏气。

(2)使用一次性吹嘴。

【思考与评价】

1. 为什么肺活量的测定要取最大值？

2. 比较肺活量与时间肺活量的意义有何不同？

【英文专业单词】

肺活量(vital capacity)

（彭碧文）

实验 18　膈神经放电

【实验目的】

(1)掌握家兔膈神经的辨认和分离；

(2)了解直接记录膈神经放电的方法。

【实验原理】

呼吸肌属于骨骼肌，其活动依赖膈神经和肋间神经的支配。脑干呼吸中枢的节律性活动通过膈神经和肋间神经下传至膈肌和肋间肌，从而产生节律性呼吸肌舒缩活动，引起呼吸运动。因此引导膈神经传出纤维的放电，可直接反映脑干呼吸中枢活动的调节。

【实验对象】

家兔。

【药品与器材】

(1)药品：20%氨基甲酸乙酯溶液、医用液体石蜡、生理盐水。

(2)器材：哺乳类动物手术器械、兔手术台、气管插管、注射器、生物机能实验系统、纱布、棉线、引导电极。

【方法与步骤】

1. 手术

(1)麻醉和固定：用20%氨基甲酸乙酯，按1g/kg体重(5ml/kg体重)的剂量从兔耳缘静脉缓慢注入，待动物麻醉后，取仰卧位将兔固定于兔手术台上。剪去颈部、剑突的毛。

(2)插气管插管：沿颈部正中切开皮肤，用止血钳钝性分离气管，在气管上做一倒"T"字形剪口，插入Y形气管插管，用棉线将气管插管结扎固定。气管插管的两个侧管各连接一根3cm长的橡皮管。

(3)分离迷走神经：在颈部分离出两侧迷走神经，在神经下穿线备用。手术完毕后用温热生理盐水纱布覆盖手术伤口部位。

(4)分离膈神经：膈神经由第4、5颈神经丛的腹支会合而成。先将动物头颈略倾向对侧，用止血钳在术侧颈外静脉与胸锁乳突肌之间向深处分离直至见到粗大横行的臂

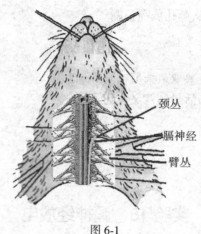

颈丛

膈神经

臂丛

图 6-1

丛神经丛。在臂丛的内侧有一条较细的由颈 4、5 脊神经分出的如细线般的神经分支，即为膈神经。膈神经横过臂丛神经并和它交叉，向后内侧行走，贴在前斜角肌腹缘表面，与气管平行进入胸腔。用玻璃分针在臂丛上方分离膈神经 2~3cm，穿线备用(图 6-1)。

(5)膈神经放电的记录：用止血钳夹住切口皮肤及组织，向上方牵引固定，使之形成皮兜。在皮兜内滴加 37℃液体石蜡保温防止神经干燥。然后用玻璃分针将膈神经轻轻挑入引导电极上，调节紧张度，神经不可牵拉过紧，记录电极应悬空，避免接触周围组织。在颈部皮肤切口处用导线使动物接地。

2. 系统的连接

引导电极连至 RM6240 生物系统第 2 通道上，记录膈神经放电。

【实验项目】

(1)待动物呼吸状态稳定后，描记正常的膈神经放电曲线。伴随呼吸节律膈神经群集放电呈梭形，电位幅度为 100~200μV。从监听器可听到与呼吸节律一致的节律性放电声音。

(2)剪断双侧迷走神经对膈神经放电的影响。剪断一侧迷走神经，观察膈神经放电变化；剪断另一侧迷走神经，观察膈神经放电变化。

【注意事项】

(1)气管插管时，应注意止血，并将气管分泌物清理干净。气管插管的侧管上的夹子在呼吸运动实验过程中不能更动，以便比较实验前、后呼吸运动和胸膜腔内压曲线的幅度变化。分离神经的操作要轻柔，分离要干净、不要让凝血块或组织块粘着在神经上

(2)若气温暖和，可不作皮兜。改用温液体石蜡条覆盖在神经上。

(3)引导电极尽量放在膈神经头端，以便神经有损伤时可将电极移向心端。注意动物和仪器的接地要可靠，以避免电磁干扰对实验结果的影响。

(4)膈神经放电的观察系指群集放电的频率、振幅。

【思考与评价】

膈神经在肺牵张反射中起什么作用？为什么？

【英文专业单词】

膈神经(phrenic nerve)

（彭碧文）

实验 19 胸内负压与气胸

【实验目的】

(1)验证胸膜腔负压的存在；

(2)学习胸膜腔内压力(胸内压)的测量方法。

【实验原理】

胸膜腔是一个密闭的腔隙，胸膜腔内的压力即为胸膜腔内压，也称胸内压，是肺内压与肺弹性回缩力之差。平静呼吸时，胸膜腔内压随呼吸运动而变化，吸气时增大，呼气时降低，但始终低于大气压力，故称胸膜腔负压。在紧闭口鼻用力呼气时，胸内压可高于大气压。在胸膜腔与外界大气相通后，当外界空气进入胸膜腔而形成气胸时，此时胸内压便与大气压相等不再呈现负压。

胸内压通常低于大气压，称为胸内负压。平静呼吸时，胸内压随呼气和吸气而升降。如果因创伤或其他原因使胸膜腔与大气相通，形成开放性气胸，胸内压与大气压相等，肺随之萎缩。

【实验对象】

家兔。

【药品与器材】

哺乳类动物手术器械、兔手术台、胸内套管或粗针头，U 形水压计，气管插管

【方法与步骤】

1. 胸内负压

(1)麻醉和固定：用20%氨基甲酸乙酯，按1g/kg 体重(5ml/kg 体重)的剂量从兔耳缘静脉缓慢注入，待动物麻醉后，取仰卧位将兔固定于兔手术台上。剪去颈部、剑突的毛。

(2)插气管插管：沿颈部正中切开皮肤，用止血钳钝性分离气管，在气管上做一倒"T"字形剪口，插入 Y 形气管插管，用棉线将气管插管结扎固定。气管插管的两个侧管各连接一根 3cm 长的橡皮管。

(3)将右侧胸部的毛剪干净，于右侧胸部腋前线第四、五肋间肋骨(左侧地 4、5 肋软骨后方的三角区称为心包区，此区前并无胸膜覆盖。)上缘垂直刺入粗针头(可先用手术刀划破皮肤后再插粗针头，切口不宜过大)，若插入胸膜腔内，则见水检压计的浮标偏离零位线而下移。(由于胸膜腔压力小于大气压)

2. 气胸

(1)沿第七肋骨走向切开胸壁皮肤(第七肋骨处为胸膜下缘，便于控制切口大小)。

(2)用止血钳分离肋间肌，造成一长约 1cm 贯穿胸壁创口，使胸膜腔与大气相通而

造成气胸。

【实验项目】

(1)平静呼吸时记录胸膜腔内压。记录平静呼吸运动,对照胸膜腔内压曲线,比较吸气和呼气时的胸膜腔内压,记录胸膜腔内压数值。

(2)深呼吸时的胸膜腔内压。将气管插管的一侧橡皮管夹闭,另一侧橡皮管再连接一根长约50cm的橡皮管,以增大无效腔,观察记录胸膜腔内压。

(3)憋气时的胸膜腔内压。在吸气末和呼气末,分别夹闭气管插管两侧管。此时处于憋气状态,观察记录胸膜腔内压。(尤其观察用力呼吸时胸膜腔内压是否高于大气压)

(4)气胸时的胸膜腔内压。观察胸膜腔内压的变化。

【注意事项】

(1)切开胸壁时的切口不宜过大,动作要迅速,避免空气漏入胸膜腔过多。

(2)形成气胸后可迅速封闭创口,并抽出胸膜腔内的气体,此时胸膜腔内压可重新出现负压。

(3)若测不到胸内负压,首先检查插管内是否有异物堵塞;并检查插管的深度,若过深将穿过胸膜进入肺组织。

(4)插管时粗针头的斜面应贴着肺组织。

【思考与评价】

1. 胸膜腔负压是如何形成的?

2. 气胸后家兔的呼吸运动如何变化?

【英文专业单词】

胸膜内压(intrapleural pressure)   气胸(pneumothorax)

(彭碧文)

实验 20　呼吸运动的调节

【实验目的】

(1)掌握家兔气管插管、呼吸运动记录等基本的手术方法;

(2)观察并分析肺牵张反射以及影响呼吸运动的各种因素。

【实验原理】

(1)人体及高等动物的呼吸运动之所以能持续地节律性地进行,是在中枢神经系统参与下,通过多种传入冲动的作用,反射性调节呼吸的频率和深度来完成的。体内、外的各种刺激,可以直接作用于中枢或通过外周感受器,反射性地影响呼吸运动,以适应机体代谢的需要。肺牵张反射是保证呼吸运动节律的机制之一。

(2)血液中CO_2的改变,通过对中枢性与外周性化学感受器的刺激及反射性调节,是保证血液中气体分压稳定的重要机制。

【实验对象】

家兔。

【药品与器材】

(1)药品：20%氨基甲酸乙酯溶液、医用液体石蜡、3%乳酸溶液、CO_2球囊、生理盐水。

(2)哺乳类动物手术器械、兔手术台、气管插管、注射器(20ml、5ml各1支)、50cm长橡皮管一根、生物机能实验系统、张力换能器、纱布、棉线、引导电极、碳酸钠钙瓶。

【方法与步骤】

1. 手术

(1)麻醉和固定：用20%氨基甲酸乙酯，按1g/kg体重(5ml/kg体重)的剂量从兔耳缘静脉缓慢注入，待动物麻醉后，取仰卧位将兔固定于兔手术台上。剪去颈部、剑突的毛。

(2)插气管插管：沿颈部正中切开皮肤，用止血钳钝性分离气管，在气管上做一倒"T"字形剪口，插入"Y"形气管插管，用棉线将气管插管结扎固定。气管插管的两个侧管各连接一根3cm长的橡皮管。

(3)分离迷走神经：在颈部分离出两侧迷走神经，在神经下穿线备用。手术完毕后用温热生理盐水纱布覆盖手术伤口部位。

(4)游离膈肌小叶：切开胸骨下端剑突部位的皮肤，并沿腹白线切开约2cm，打开腹腔。用纱布轻轻将内脏沿膈肌向下压；暴露出剑突软骨和剑突骨柄，辨认剑突，其内侧面附着的两块膈小肌，仔细分离剑突与膈小肌之间的组织，于膈肌小叶背后穿线打结并和张力换能器相连接。

2. 系统的连接

张力换能器连接到RM6240生物系统第1通道上，记录呼吸运动曲线。

【实验项目】

(1)描记对照曲线：待动物呼吸状态稳定后，描记呼吸运动曲线。

(2)吸入气中CO_2浓度增加的影响：将充有CO_2的球囊导气管口对准气管插管逐渐松开螺旋夹，气袋加压，使兔吸入气CO_2浓度升高，观察呼吸运动变化。

(3)吸入气中O_2浓度降低的影响：将充有N_2的球囊导气管口对准气管插管逐渐松开螺旋夹，气袋加压，使兔吸入O_2浓度降低，观察对呼吸运动的影响。

(4)增大呼吸无效腔：将气管插管的一侧管夹闭，把30cm长的橡皮管连在气管插管的另一侧上，动物通过此橡皮管进行呼吸。观察对呼吸运动的影响。

(5)增加气道阻力：夹闭气管插管其中一侧的橡皮管，用手或止血钳压住另一侧橡皮管，观察对呼吸运动的影响。

(6)增加血液酸碱度：自兔耳缘静脉注入3%乳酸1~2ml，观察对呼吸运动影响。

(7)颈迷走神经在呼吸运动调节的作用：记录一段对照呼吸曲线后，先切断一侧迷走神经，观察呼吸运动的变化。再切断另一侧迷走神经，观察呼吸运动的变化(包括频率和深度)。然后，以电刺激(刺激参数：连续刺激、强度为3V左右、波宽为1~2ms)，刺激一侧迷走神经的中枢端10s左右，观察刺激期间呼吸运动的变化。

（8）肺扩张反射现象观察：在观察一段正常呼吸运动后，于一次呼吸的吸气相之末，将气管插管的一侧管（呼吸通气的侧管）连接30ml注射器（内装有20ml空气），堵塞插管的另一侧管口，同时将注射器内的20ml空气迅速注入肺内，使肺维持在扩张状态，观察呼吸运动和膈神经放电的变化。出现明显效应后立即放开堵塞口。

【注意事项】

（1）气管插管时，应注意止血，并将气管分泌物清理干净。气管插管的侧管上的夹子在呼吸运动实验过程中不能移动，以便比较实验前、后呼吸运动和胸膜腔内压曲线的幅度变化。每项观察项目前均应有正常描记曲线作为对照。每项观察时间不宜过长，出现效应后应立即去掉施加因素，待呼吸运动恢复正常后再进行下一项观察。

（2）经耳缘静脉注射乳酸时，注意不要刺穿静脉，以免乳酸外漏，引起动物躁动。

（3）电极刺激迷走神经向中枢端之前，一定要调整好刺激强度，以免因刺激强度过强而造成动物全身肌肉紧张，发生屏气，影响实验结果。

【思考与评价】

1. 平静呼吸时，如何确定呼吸运动曲线与吸气和呼气运动的对应关系？比较吸气、呼气、憋气时的胸膜腔内压，读出胸膜腔内压数值。

2. CO_2增多、低O_2和乳酸增多对呼吸运动有何影响？其作用途径有何不同？

3. 在平静呼吸时，胸膜腔内压为何始终低于大气压？在什么情况下胸膜腔内压可高于大气压？

4. 切断两侧迷走神经前、后呼吸运动有何变化？迷走神经在节律性呼吸运动中起什么作用？

【英文专业单词】

肺牵张反射 pulmonary stretch reflex

（万曙霞）

实验21　离体小肠平滑肌标本制备与各种因素对小肠平滑肌活动的影响

【实验目的】

（1）学习哺乳动物离体器官或组织灌流的实验方法。

（2）观察哺乳动物小肠平滑肌的一般特性及药物对离体小肠平滑肌的作用。

【实验原理】

哺乳动物的胃肠平滑肌（gastrointestinal smooth muscle）具有较低的兴奋性（excitability），缓慢的收缩性（contractility），不规则的自动节律性（autorhythmicity）、较大的伸展性（extensibility）、持续的紧张性（tonicity）和对理化刺激较敏感而对电刺激不敏感等生理特性。这些特性对维持消化管的一定压力，保持胃肠等的一定形态和位置，适合于消化管内食物的消化具有生理意义。

【实验对象】

家兔。

【实验药品与器材】

1. 药品：1∶10 000(g/ml)肾上腺素、1∶100 000 乙酰胆碱(g/m1)、1∶10 000(g/ml)阿托品、1%CaCl₂溶液、1mol/L(pH=1) 盐酸、1mol/L NaOH、台氏液。

2. 器材：RM6240C 或 BL-420E 生物信号采集系统、离体平滑肌灌流恒温装置、温度计、哺乳动物手术器械一套、兔手术台、铁支架、烧杯、滴管。

【实验方法与步骤】

1. 恒温平滑肌浴槽的准备

实验前先将自来水注满浴槽，然后将台氏液加入预液管和药液管(即标本槽，加入台氏液到浴槽高度的 2/3 处)。恒温工作点定在 38℃左右，开启升温开关，搅拌轮转动，加热器通电加热至所需温度，可采用外加温度计调整药液管内温度到 37℃。打开供氧开关，即可产生空气泡供氧，调节微调旋钮使气泡一个一个地冒出，不能过快以免液面振动而影响记录。肌槽的右侧面有与预液管、药液管相通的出液管，用弹簧夹控制出液量(图 6-2)

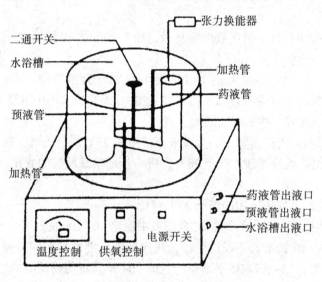

图 6-2　恒温平滑肌浴槽

2. 离体小肠平滑肌标本的制备

用木槌击兔头致昏，快速打开腹腔，以胃幽门与十二指肠交界处为起点，沿肠缘剪去肠系膜，剪取长 10~15cm 的十二指肠管。置于 4℃台氏液中轻轻漂洗。实验时剪取 2~3cm 的肠段(靠近头段)，用棉线结扎肠段两端，一端系于药液槽内的标本固定钩上，另一端与张力换能器相连。适当调节换能器的高度，使标本与换能器的连线松紧合适，正好悬挂在药液管中央，避免与药液管的管壁接触。

3. 仪器连接与设置

将张力换能器信号输入端连接 RM6240C 或 BL-420E 生物信号采集系统。开机进入实验操作系统，调整走纸速度，基线及有关参数。

【实验项目】

(1)描记一段小肠平滑肌正常收缩曲线，注意观察小肠平滑肌的紧张性、收缩的幅度和节律。收缩曲线基线的高低表示小肠平滑肌紧张性的高低，收缩曲线的幅度大小表示小肠平滑肌收缩活动的强弱。

(2)肾上腺素的作用：用滴管加 1~2 滴 1∶10 000 肾上腺素于药液管中，观察收缩曲线的节律、波形和幅度有无改变。待观察到明显作用后，先打开药液管的出口放弃含肾上腺素的台氏液，再打开二通开关使预液管预温的台氏液通向药液管，如此重复冲洗3 次，以洗涤或稀释残留的肾上腺素，使达到无效浓度。换入等量的台氏液，待平滑肌收缩恢复后，再进行下一项观察。

(3)乙酰胆碱的作用：按上述方法加 1~2 滴 1∶100 000 乙酰胆碱于药液管中，观察收缩曲线的变化，效果明显后，按上述方法冲洗。

(4)阿托品的作用：在药液管中加入 1∶10 000 的阿托品 2~4 滴，2 min 后，再加1∶100 000 乙酰胆碱 1~2 滴。观察收缩曲线的变化，并与(3)的实验结果比较有何不同。冲洗方法同上。

(5)$CaCl_2$ 的作用：待平滑肌收缩恢复后，加 1% $CaCl_2$ 溶液 1~2 滴于药液管内，观察平滑肌收缩活动的反应。

(6)酸碱的作用：加 1 mol/L 的 HCl 溶液 1~2 滴于药液管内，观察平滑肌的反应，在加 HCl 使平滑肌收缩活动明显改变的基础上加 1mol/L 的 NaOH 溶液 1~2 滴于药液管内，观察平滑肌的反应。冲洗方法同上。

(7)温度的影响：将药液管中的台氏液全部换成 25℃ 的台氏液，观察小肠平滑肌的收缩活动有何变化。然后逐渐加温至 38℃，进一步观察其反应的变化。

【注意事项】

(1)必须预先准备好更换用的新鲜 37℃ 台氏液。

(2)标本安装好后，应在新鲜 37℃ 台氏液中稳定 10~20min。

(3)药液管内的台氏液必需没过肠段，每次换液后液面均应保持同一高度，并保持药液管恒温为 38℃，以免影响肠平滑肌的收缩功能及其对药物反应的稳定性。

(4)实验中始终要通入空气，气泡不要太多，以每秒 2~3 个为宜。

(5)每个实验项目结束后，应立即用 37℃ 台氏液冲洗，待肠段活动恢复正常后，再进行下一个实验项目。

(6)实验过程中要防止一次性加药过量，以免引起不可逆反应。

(7)各试剂的滴管要专用，避免相互污染。

【思考题】

1. 制备小肠平滑肌标本时，为什么要取小肠上段，尤其是十二指肠段的平滑肌?

2. 哺乳类动物离体器官和组织在灌流液中保持良好状态需具备哪些基本灌流条件?

3. 上述各种因素对小肠平滑肌收缩活动有何影响? 为什么?

4. 比较肾上腺素、乙酰胆碱对小肠平滑肌和心肌的作用有何不同?

5. 制备小肠平滑肌标本时,为什么不用麻醉后的兔小肠,而用击昏兔的小肠?

【英文专业单词】

胃肠平滑肌(gastrointestinal smooth muscle)　兴奋性(excitability)

收缩性(contractility)　　　　　　　　　　自动节律性(autorhythmicity)

伸展性(extensibility)　　　　　　　　　　紧张性(tonicity)

(严晓红)

实验 22　胃肠运动的观察

【实验目的】

本实验的目的是了解哺乳类动物胃和小肠运动的形式及神经、体液因素对胃肠运动的调节。

【实验原理】

食物的消化包括机械性消化和化学性消化。前者是通过消化道运动,主要指胃肠运动(gastrointestinal motility)即胃和小肠平滑肌机械性收缩与舒张实现的。其中胃运动的基本形式呈紧张性收缩(tonic contraction)、容受性舒张(receptive relaxation)及蠕动(peristalsis);小肠运动形式主要为分节运动(segmentation contraction)、蠕动。在体内胃肠平滑肌受神经系统支配及体液因素的影响。

胃肠运动的神经调节受自主神经和肠神经系统的调节。胃肠道拥有自己的局部神经系统,称为肠神经系统。它们由大量神经元、神经纤维以及自主神经纤维组成。肠神经系统含有肾上腺素能、胆碱能及分泌其他神经递质的神经元。

自主神经系统也称外来神经系统,包括交感神经(sympathetic nerve)和副交感神经(parasympathetic nerve)。交感神经兴奋时,节后神经纤维释放去甲肾上腺素(noradrenalin,NA),与平滑肌膜上 α、β 受体结合,产生抑制效应,使胃肠运动减弱;副交感神经兴奋时,其节后纤维释放神经递质(neurotransmitter)乙酰胆碱(acetylcholin,Ach)与平滑肌膜上 M 受体结合,产生兴奋效应,使胃肠运动增强。

【实验对象】

家兔。

【实验药品与器材】

(1)药品:20%氨基甲酸乙酯、台氏液(或生理盐水)、1∶10 000 肾上腺素、新斯的明(neostigmine,1mg/ml)、1∶10 000 乙酰胆碱、阿托品(atropin,0.5mg/ml)。

(2)器材:RM6240C 或 BL-420E 生物信号采集系统、刺激输出线、保护电极、哺乳动物手术器械一套、兔手术台、玻璃分针、纱布、线、注射器(20ml 和 1ml)、注射针头。

【实验方法与步骤】

1. 家兔的麻醉、固定与备皮

由耳缘静脉注射 20%氨基甲酸乙酯(1g/kg),待兔麻醉后,背位固定于兔手术台上，剪去颈部和上腹部手术野的兔毛。

2. 手术步骤

(1)气管插管：颈部正中皮肤切口 4~5cm，剪开筋膜，钝性分离颈部肌肉，暴露气管，穿索线备用；于甲状软骨下 1cm 左右的气管软骨环上行倒"T"字形切口，朝心脏方向插入气管插管并用备用索线结扎固定插管。

(2)于剑突下 0.5cm 左右，沿正中线切开腹部皮肤 8~10cm，暴露胃、肠。

(3)分离膈下迷走神经：用玻璃分针于膈下食管末端分离左侧迷走神经的前支 1~2cm，穿丝线备用。

(4)分离内脏大神经：于左侧腹后壁肾上腺的上方找到内脏大神经，分离出 1~2cm，穿线备用。

3. 仪器连接

连接保护电极于 RM6240C 或 BL-420E 生物信号采集系统的刺激输出线，开机进入实验操作系统。

【实验项目】

(1)正常情况下的胃肠运动：未给予任何刺激情况下观察胃肠运动形式(紧张度、蠕动、逆蠕动、小肠分节运动等)。

(2)用保护电极连续电脉冲刺激(刺激强度为 2~5V；波宽为 0.2ms；刺激频率为 20~30Hz)膈下迷走神经 1~3min，观察胃肠运动的变化。

(3)待胃肠运动恢复正常后，先从耳缘静脉注射阿托品 0.25mg/kg，再用连续电脉冲刺激膈下迷走神经，观察胃肠运动的变化。

(4)耳缘静脉注射拟胆碱药新斯的明 0.1~0.2mg，观察胃肠运动的变化。

(5)于耳缘静脉注射肾上腺素(1∶10 000)0.3~0.5ml，观察胃肠运动的变化。

(6)于耳缘静脉注射乙酰胆碱(1∶10 000)0.3~0.5ml，观察胃肠运动的变化。

(7)用上述 2 的方法刺激内脏大神经 1~3min，观察胃肠运动的变化。

【注意事项】

(1)腹部切口须沿正中线进行，此处为腹直肌鞘所在，可避免出血。

(2)整个实验过程中，为避免胃肠暴露时间过长，使腹腔内温度下降和小肠表面干燥，影响胃肠运动，必须经常用温热的生理盐水湿润。天气寒冷时要注意保温。

(3)实验动物须在实验前 1h 喂饱，或服用 5%硫酸钠 10ml。

(4)实验时，不要过度牵拉胃肠。

(5)每完成一个实验项目后，间隔数分钟待胃肠运动恢复后再进行下一个实验项目。

【思考题】

1. 兔的胃肠运动有哪些形式？如何观察？

2. 如何分离膈下迷走神经和内脏大神经？

3. 电刺激迷走神经和内脏大神经时，胃肠运动会出现与预期结果相反的现象吗？为什么？

【英文专业单词】

胃肠运动(gastrointestinal motility)　　紧张性收缩(tonic contraction)

容受性舒张(receptive relaxation)　　蠕动(peristalsis)

分节运动(segmentation contraction)　　副交感神经(parasympathetic nerve)

交感神经(sympathetic nerve)　　乙酰胆碱(acetylcholin，Ach)

去甲肾上腺素(noradrenalin，NA)

(严晓红)

第7章 消化生理

实验23 家兔胆汁分泌的调节

【实验目的】

(1)学习并掌握胆总管插管技术与胆汁引流的方法。

(2)以胆汁的量为指标,观察神经与体液因素对胆汁分泌的调控。

【实验原理】

肝细胞分泌胆汁是一个连续的过程。在非消化期,由于奥迪氏括约肌收缩阻止胆汁排入十二指肠,肝细胞分泌的胆汁主要流入胆囊内进行储存和浓缩;在消化期,奥迪氏括约肌舒张,肝细胞新分泌的胆汁(肝胆汁)与储存于胆囊内的胆汁(胆囊胆汁)均可排入十二指肠腔,参与脂类物质的消化与吸收。胆汁分泌与排出受多种因素的调控,其中,食物是引起胆汁分泌和排出的自然刺激物;迷走神经兴奋既可促进肝胆汁的分泌,也可促进胆囊胆汁的排出;促胃液素、胰泌素、缩胆囊素、胆盐等均可促进胆汁分泌与排出;小肠内 pH 值降低可刺激胰泌素的释放进而促进胆汁的分泌与排出。

【实验对象】

家兔(实验前喂食),体重 2~2.5kg。

【实验药品与器材】

(1)药品:20%氨基甲酸乙酯溶液或 3%戊巴比妥钠溶液、0.9%生理盐水、1∶10 000乙酰胆碱、0.1mol/L 稀盐酸。

(2)器材:RM6240 生物信号采集系统,哺乳动物手术器械,气管插管,细塑料插管,记滴器,刺激电极,20ml、5ml、1ml 注射器,针头,酒精灯,培养皿,手术灯,纱布,棉绳,丝线,铁支架,双凹夹,兔手术台。

【实验方法及步骤】

1. 动物手术

(1)麻醉与固定:称重后按由家兔耳缘静脉缓慢注入 20%氨基甲酸乙酯(1g/kg)或 3%戊巴比妥钠(30~40mg/kg)以麻醉动物,随后将家兔仰卧位固定于兔手术台上。

(2)气管插管:剪去颈部手术野被毛,行颈部手术以暴露气管并进行气管插管。

(3)胆总管插管:①剪去上腹部手术野被毛;②自剑突入沿正中线向下做 7~10cm 长皮肤切口,再沿腹白线剪开腹壁和腹膜(勿损伤腹腔脏器),暴露胃和肝;③在膈下食管末端前壁外膜下,用玻璃分针分离出迷走神经的前支 1cm,穿一丝线备用;④将肝轻轻向上翻起，找到胆囊后用动脉夹夹闭胆囊管，用注射器抽出 1ml 胆汁备用；⑤将胃轻轻拉出，在十二指肠上端背面肠壁找到一略微隆起的十二指肠乳头(胆总管十二指肠入口)；⑥用玻璃分针分离末段胆总管约 1cm，穿一丝线备用；⑦在十二指乳头处用眼科剪剪一小口，将细塑料插管插入胆总管内，可见黄绿色胆汁流出，将胆总管与插管一起结扎并固定；⑧术毕，用温热生理盐水纱布覆盖手术创口。

2. 仪器连接

调整塑料插管与记滴器的位置，使从塑料插管流出的胆汁正好同时落在记滴器的受滴电极上。将液滴信号引导线接 1 号通道输入插座。

【实验项目】

(1)记录未经任何处理因素情况下家兔的胆汁排出量。

(2)用保护电极以中等强度的脉冲电流(刺激强度为 5～10V，刺激频率为 20～30Hz)连续刺激迷走神经 1min、间隔 2min，再重复刺激 2 次，观察胆汁分泌的潜伏期和分泌量。

(3)经耳缘静脉注射 1∶10 000 乙酰胆碱 0.5ml，观察胆汁分泌的潜伏期和分泌量。

(4)先经耳缘静脉注射生理盐水 5ml 作为对照，再注射稀释的胆汁(1ml 胆汁用生理盐水稀释 10 倍)5ml，观察胆汁分泌的潜伏期和分泌量。

(5)结扎十二指肠胃端与空肠端后，向十二指肠腔内注射 37℃ 0.1mol/L 稀盐酸 20ml，观察胆汁分泌的潜伏期和分泌量。

【注意事项】

(1)分离胆总管时须十分小心，以防损伤伴行的血管。

(2)胆总管壁薄，实验过程中谨防管壁被刺破或胆总管扭曲导致胆汁引流不畅。

(3)术毕应用温热生理盐水浸湿的纱布覆盖以给家兔保温保湿。

(4)后一项实验项目须待前一项目作用基本消失后方能进行。

【思考题】

1. 刺激膈下迷走神经与静脉注射乙酰胆碱引起胆汁分泌的潜伏期和分泌量有何不同？

2. 静脉注射稀释的胆汁通过何种机制促进胆汁的分泌？

【英文专业单词】

胆汁分泌(bile seeretion)

(陈桃香)

第8章 泌尿生理

实验24 尿液生成的影响因素

【实验目的】

(1)学习并掌握膀胱或输尿管插管技术。

(2)以尿量和尿质为指标,观察各种因素对尿生成的影响并分析其作用机制。

【实验原理】

尿液的生成包括:①肾小球的滤过;②肾小管和集合管的重吸收;③肾小管和集合管的分泌等三个基本过程。任何影响这些过程的因素都会引起尿液量或质的变化。

【实验对象】

家兔,体重2~2.5kg。

【实验药品与器材】

(1)药品:20%氨基甲酸乙酯溶液或3%戊巴比妥钠溶液、50%葡萄糖溶液、0.9%生理盐水、1:10 000去甲肾上腺素、垂体后叶素、呋塞米(速尿)、0.6%酚红注射液,10% NaOH、肝素、尿糖试纸。

(2)器材:RM6240生物信号采集系统,压力换能器,哺乳动物手术器械,膀胱插管或输尿管插管,动脉插管,细塑料插管,记滴器,动脉夹,刺激电极,20ml、10ml、5ml、1ml注射器,针头,试管,试管架,酒精灯,培养皿,手术灯,纱布,棉绳,丝线,兔手术台。

【实验方法及步骤】

1. 动物手术

(1)麻醉与固定:称重后由家兔耳缘静脉缓慢注入20%氨基甲酸乙酯(1g/kg)或3%戊巴比妥钠(30~40mg/kg)以麻醉动物,随后将家兔仰卧位固定于兔手术台上。

(2)气管插管与动脉插管:剪去颈部手术野被毛,行颈部手术以暴露气管并进行气管插管,然后分别分离左侧颈总动脉与右侧迷走神经(穿一丝线备用)。动脉插管:从左侧颈总动脉下方穿两根丝线,先用一根丝线结扎左侧颈总动脉远心端,用动脉夹夹住近心端,然后在结扎处下部剪一小斜口,插入充满肝素化生理盐水的动脉插管,用另一丝线结扎固定。松开动脉夹,记录动脉血压。

(3)收集尿液:可选择膀胱导尿法或输尿管导尿法。剪去下腹部手术野被毛。在耻骨联合上缘沿正中线向上做5cm长皮肤切口,再沿腹白线剪开腹壁和腹膜(勿损伤腹腔脏器），暴露膀胱，并轻轻地将其翻转至腹腔外以暴露膀胱三角区。在膀胱底部找到两侧输尿管，认清其在膀胱开口的部位。

（4）膀胱插管：在两侧输尿管的下方穿一丝线，将膀胱上翻，结扎尿道。然后在膀胱壁血管较少处做一荷包缝合，保留荷包两端缝线。在荷包中央膀胱壁剪一小口，插入充满生理盐水浸泡过的膀胱插管，收紧荷包两端缝线并结扎固定膀胱插管。术毕，用温热生理盐水浸泡过的纱布覆盖手术创口。调整膀胱插管另一端与记滴器的位置，使从膀胱插管流出的尿液正好同时落在记滴器的受滴电极上。

（5）输尿管插管：将输尿管与周围组织轻轻分离，在每侧输尿管下方各穿两根丝线。首先用一根丝线将一侧输尿管近膀胱端扎住（使尿液不能流进膀胱），然后在结扎处上部剪一"V"字形小口，向肾脏方向插入充满生理盐水的输尿管插管，用另一根丝线将输尿管插管与输尿管扎紧并固定。用同样的方法插入另一侧输尿管导管，并结扎固定。术毕，用温热生理盐水浸泡的纱布覆盖手术创口。调整输尿管插管另一端与记滴器的位置，使从输尿管插管流出的尿液正好同时落在记滴器的受滴电极上。

2. 仪器连接

将液滴信号引导线接 1 号通道输入插座，压力换能器接 2 号通道输入插座。

【实验项目】

（1）记录未经任何处理因素情况下家兔的动脉血压曲线和尿量。

（2）从耳缘静脉快速（1min 内）注射 37℃生理盐水 30ml，观察血压和尿量的变化。

（3）从耳缘静脉注射 1∶10 000 去甲肾上腺素 0.3~0.5ml，观察血压和尿量的变化。

（4）取尿液两滴，用尿糖试纸测定尿糖。然后从耳缘静脉注射 50%葡萄糖溶液 2ml，观察血压和尿量的变化。待尿量明显增加时，再取尿液 2 滴作尿糖定性试验。

（5）从耳缘静脉注射垂体后叶素 2U，观察血压和尿量的变化。

（6）从耳缘静脉注射呋塞米（5mg/kg），观察血压和尿量的变化。

（7）静脉注射 0.6%酚红溶液 0.5ml，并开始计时，用盛有 10%NaOH 溶液的培养皿收集尿滴。如果尿中有酚红排出，遇 NaOH 则显紫红色。计算从注射酚红起到尿中排出酚红所需要的时间（如果输尿管或膀胱插管过长，要考虑尿液流过的时间）。

（8）电刺激迷走神经：结扎并剪断右侧迷走神经，用保护电极以中等强度的脉冲电流（刺激强度为 5~10V，刺激频率为 20~50Hz）间断刺激其外周端，观察血压和尿量的变化。

（9）分离一侧股动脉，插入塑料导管进行控制放血，使动脉血压迅速下降至 50mmHg 左右，观察尿量的变化。再迅速补充生理盐水，观察血压和尿量的变化。

【注意事项】

（1）实验前给家兔多喂青菜，以保证家兔在实验中有充足的尿液排出。

（2）本实验需多次经耳缘静脉给药，应注意保护家兔耳缘静脉。

（3）依次进行实验项目，后一项实验项目须待前一项目作用基本消失，血压与尿量基本恢复后方能进行。

（4）实验项目的安排顺序是：在尿量多的基础上实施减少尿量的实验项目；在尿量少的基础上进行促进尿生成的实验项目。

（5）注射 50% 葡萄糖溶液后，应用新的容器来收集尿液，以便做尿糖测定（如不更换容器，也可将尿液直接滴在尿糖试纸上）。

（6）电刺激迷走神经观察尿量变化时，强度应适宜；勿用强电流连续刺激。

（7）在寒冬季节，要注意给动物保温。

【思考题】

1. 本实验中影响肾小球滤过的因素有哪些？影响肾小管和集合管重吸收与分泌的因素有哪些？

2. 电刺激迷走神经如何影响尿量？

【英文专业单词】

尿生成（urine formation）

（陈桃香）

第9章 感觉器官生理

实验 25 视敏度测定

【实验目的】

(1)通过正确使用视力表、掌握视敏度的定义;

(2)掌握视敏度、色觉的测定方法。

【实验原理】

眼辨别物体形态细节的能力称为视敏度(visual acuity),又叫视力,它表示视觉分辨物体细节的能力。通常是以能辨别两条平行光线的最小距离为衡量标准。视敏度由物体的视角所决定,即物体最边沿两点与眼睛的角膜所形成的夹角,它等于视觉所能分辨的以角度分为单位的视角的倒数。一般是以观察一定距离处的视力表上的视标("E"的开口)来确定视力的。被测试者在视力表前5m处若能分辨一个1分视角的视标开口,则视力定为1。影响视敏度的因素很多,例如,视象离视网膜中央凹越近视敏度越高,中央凹的视敏度最高;物体的照明水平提高,视敏度也增加;在一定照明水平上,物体与背景的对比度增加,视敏度也随之提高。

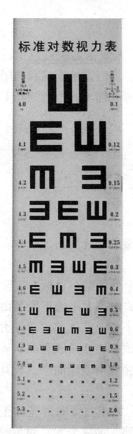

图 9-1 标准对数视力表

【实验对象】

人。

【实验药品与材料】

标准对数视力表。

【实验项目】

视敏度的测定。

【实验方法】

视敏度的测定:

将如图 9-1 所示标准视力表挂在光线充足而均匀的墙上,表上第 11 行字与受检者眼睛在同一高度。

受检者站立或坐在视力表前 5m 处,用遮眼板遮住一眼,一般先测右眼,后测左眼。

检查者用指示棒从上而下逐行指点，每指一字，令受检者说出或以手势表示字母缺口朝向，直到完全不能辨别为止。此时受检者能看清的最后一行字母的表旁数值即为该眼的视力。

【注意事项】

检测过程中应严格控制读图时间，不可长时间思考。

【思考与评价】

标准对数视力表上的数字代表什么意义？

【英文专业单词】

视敏度（visual acuity）

（彭碧文）

实验 26　视觉调节与瞳孔对光反射

【实验目的】

应用球面镜成像规律，证明在视近物时眼折光系统的调节主要是晶状体前表面凸度的增加，并观察视近物时和光刺激时瞳孔缩小的现象。

【实验原理】

观察视觉调节反射与瞳孔对光反射（pupillary light reflex）。人眼由远视近或由近视远时都会发生调节反射。当由远视近时，引起晶状体凸度增加，同时发生缩瞳和两眼辐辏；由近视远时，即发生相反的变化。人眼在受到光刺激时，瞳孔缩小，称为瞳孔对光反射。

【实验对象】

人。

【实验药品与器材】

蜡烛、火柴、电筒。

【实验项目】

观察者与受试者在暗室内进行实验，观察视觉调节反射与瞳孔对光反射。

【方法与步骤】

（1）点燃的蜡烛放于受试者眼的前外方，让受试者注视数米外的某一目标。实验者可以观察到蜡烛在受试者眼内的三个烛像（图 9-2）。其中最亮的中等大小的正像是由角膜前表面反射而成；通过瞳孔可见到一个较暗而大的正立像，系由晶状体前表面反射而成；另一个较亮而最小的倒立像，则是晶状体后表面反射而形成。由于角膜和晶状体前表面均为向前的凸面，故形成正立像；晶状体前表面曲率小于角膜前表面曲率，故其像较大且暗。晶状体后表面为凹面向前，其像为倒立，且小而亮。

（2）让受试者转而注视 15cm 处的蜡烛，此时可见图中最大的正立像向最亮的正立像靠近且变小。这说明视近物时晶状体前表面凸度增加靠近角膜，曲率变大，而角膜前表面和晶状体后表面的曲率及位置均未明显改变。这就是眼的调节反射。

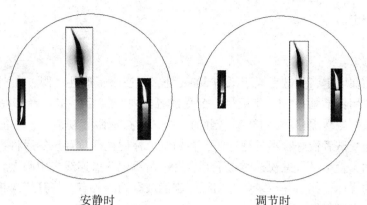

安静时　　　　　　　　　　　调节时

图 9-2　视觉调节反射进行时，眼球各反光面映像的变化

（3）在受试者注视近物时，还可见到瞳孔缩小，双眼向鼻侧会聚，前者称为缩瞳反射，后者称为辐辏反射（convergence reflex）。

（4）让受试者注视远方，观察其瞳孔大小。再用电筒照射受试者一眼，可见受光照眼瞳孔立刻缩小，如用手在鼻侧挡住以防止光照射另一眼，重复上述试验，可见双眼瞳孔同时缩小，称为互感性对光反射。

【注意事项】

（1）本实验应在暗室内进行。

（2）电筒照射受试者一眼检查瞳孔对光反射后，应休息 5min 再重复，避免眼睛疲劳。

【思考与评价】

蜡烛在受试者眼睛成像分别是如何产生的？

【英文专业单词】

瞳孔对光反射（pupillary light reflex）　辐辏反射（convergence reflex）

（彭碧文）

实验 27　生理盲点的测定

【实验原理】

视网膜上无感光细胞的部位称为盲点（blind spot）。盲点是视神经穿过的视网膜之处，无视觉细胞分布，物体的影像落在这里也不能引起视觉。

【实验对象】

人。

【药品与器材】

铅笔、直尺坐标纸等。

【实验项目】

盲点的测定。

【方法与步骤】

盲点的测定：

将白纸贴在墙上，受试者立于纸前 50cm 处，用遮眼板遮住一眼，在白纸上与另一眼平行的地方用铅笔画一"十"字记号。令受试者注视"十"字。实验者将视标由"十"字中心向被测眼颞侧缓缓移动(图 9-3)。此时，受试者被测眼直视前方，不能随视标的移动而移动。当受试者恰好看不见视标时，在白纸上标记视标位置。然后将视标继续向眼颞侧缓缓移动，直至又看见视标时记下其位置。由所记两点连线之中心点起，沿着各个方向向外移动视标，找出并记录各方向视标刚能被看到的各点，将其依次相连，即得一个椭圆形的盲点投射区。

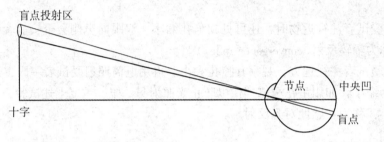

图 9-3   计算盲点的直径示意图

根据相似三角形各对应边成正比定理，可计算出盲点与中央凹的距离及盲点直径，如下公式：

$$盲点直径 = 盲点在野上直径 \times \frac{节点到视网膜(15cm)}{节点到纸(50cm)}$$

【注意事项】

(1)用单眼注视正前方不动。

(2)色标移动方向正确。

(3)生理性盲点呈椭圆形，垂直径 7.5cm±2cm，横径 5.5cm±2cm。盲点在注视中心外侧 15.5cm，在水平线下 1.5cm。

【思考与评价】

1. 试述测定盲点与中央凹的距离和盲点直径的原理。

2. 在我们日常注视物体时，为什么没有感觉到生理性盲点的存在？

3. 生理盲点的直径为多大？如果直径扩大会是什么原因造成的？

【英文专业单词】

视野(visual field)   视敏度(visual acuity)

盲点(blind spot)

（彭碧文）

实验 28 声音的传导通路

【实验目的】
(1)学习如何使用音叉产生声音；

(2)了解听觉器官的功能；

(3)了解声音传导的途径。

【实验原理】
听力丧失是由于听觉系统中任何地方的异常所产生的声音灵敏度损失。多种因素会导致听力损失。

空气传导试验是通过空气刺激耳朵，测试外耳道和中耳的功能、内耳的完整性、第八颅神经和中央听觉通路。骨传导试验使用振动音叉放置在头部，通过外耳道和中耳传导。骨传导测试可以帮助区分内耳、第八颅神经和中枢听觉传导通路的异常。

林纳试验，又称气骨导比较试验，通过比较同侧耳气导和骨导听觉时间判断耳聋的性质。

Weber 试验，又称骨导偏向试验，用于比较受试者两耳的辅导听力。

【实验对象】
人。

【实验器材】
音叉(256Hz 和 512Hz)、棉花球、橡胶锤、计时器。

【实验方法】
1. 林纳试验
将敲响的音叉柄底部先压置于受试耳的乳突部鼓窦区，测其骨导听力，直至不再听到声音，记录骨导听力时间；立即将音叉壁置于同侧外耳道口外侧，测其气导听力，直至不再听到声音，记录气导听力时间。

(1)听力正常者：气导听力时间大于骨导时间的两倍($AC>BC$)，为阳性(+)，表示受试者听力正常。

(2)感音神经性聋：气导听力时间大于骨导时间但不足两倍($AC>BC$)，为阳性(+)，表示受试者听力感音神经性聋。

(3)传导性聋：骨导听力时间大于气导听力，为阴性(−)，表示受试者听力传导性聋。

(4)混合性聋：气导与骨导时间相等(AC=BC)，为(±)，表示混合性聋。

2. 模仿传导性听力损失
用棉球堵塞外耳道，重复林纳试验。

3. Weber 测试(图 9-4)
可以使用一个 256Hz 或一个 512Hz 音叉。在这个试验中，振动音叉的柄底部，放在头部中线上的任何一点。让受试者指出声音的偏向，即哪侧或是双侧听到声音更响。

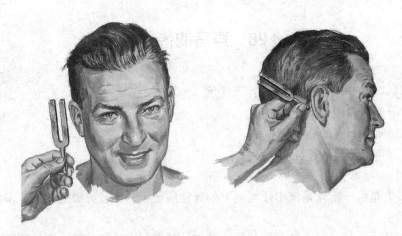

图 9-4　音叉空气传导测试正确定位(左)和骨传导(右)

（1）听力正常或双耳听损相等："＝"表示两只耳朵都听见骨导声，即听力正常或双耳听损相等。

（2）传导性聋："→患耳"表示患耳侧听见骨导声，即患耳为传导性聋。

（3）感音神经性聋："→健耳"表示健耳侧听见骨导声，即患耳为感音神经性聋。

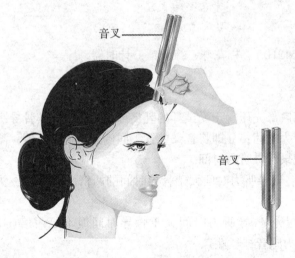

音叉

音叉

图 9-5　Weber 试验音叉的中线定位

【讨论】

1. 空气传导与骨传导的比较。

2. 传导性耳聋和感音神经性听力损失的机制是什么？

【英文专业单词】

气传导(air conduction)　骨传导(bone conduction)

（彭碧文）

实验 29　耳蜗微音器效应和微音器电位的测定

【实验目的】

本实验要求掌握盲点的定义及盲点的测定方法。

【实验内容】

观察耳蜗微音器电位和听神经动作电位的特征及其相互关系。

【实验原理】

耳蜗接受声波刺激后，能像微音器那样将声波振动的机械能转变为电能(电信号)。耳蜗的这一换能作用称为微音器效应(microphonic effect)，转换而来的电位变化，称为微音器电位(cochlear microphonic potential，CM)。CM 的波形、频率与刺激声波相符，其位相随声波位相的改变而改变，频率在 10 000Hz 以上，几乎没有潜伏期，也没有不应期，长时间刺激后，既无适应现象产生，也不发生疲劳。在温度下降、深度麻醉、甚至动物死亡后半小时内，CM 仍可出现。将引导电极放在豚鼠内耳圆窗附近，用短声刺激，能获得 CM，同时可记录到耳蜗神经动作电位，它出现于 CM 之后，一般可见 2~3 个负波(N_1、N_2、N_3)。这些负波可能是神经纤维的动作电位同步化的结果，电位的大小能反映被兴奋的神经纤维数目的多少。微音器电位经过放大器放大后输入电脑电脑多媒体声卡，通过音箱可听得与刺激声波相同的声音，此为微音器效应(microphonic effect)。

【实验对象】

豚鼠(体重 300~400g、听反应阳性)。

【实验药品与器材】

常规手术器械、小骨钻、RM6240B 生理信号采集处理系统、银球引导电极、20%氨基甲酸乙酯、温热生理盐水、纱布、棉球、注射器、豚鼠解剖台(或蛙板)、屏蔽箱。

【实验方法与步骤】

(1)用 20%氨基甲酸乙酯，按 6ml/kg 体重腹腔注射麻醉。

(2)将一侧耳廓四周的毛剪干净，沿耳廓根部的后上缘切开皮肤，分离并剔净肌肉。

(3)充分暴露颞骨乳突，该部位在枕骨粗隆下方约 1.5cm、外耳道开口后方约 0.5cm 处。用小骨钻在此钻一小孔，用镊子将骨孔稍扩展(直径约 1mm)。注意该骨质很薄，为 0.5~1mm，切勿使小骨钻插入鼓室过深而伤及耳蜗。

(4)把动物移入屏蔽箱内侧卧。将银球电极前端稍弯曲，穿过骨孔轻轻探向深部，使银球与圆窗膜接触。无关电极和接地电极插入切口皮下。引导电极输入端与生物信号采集系统通道 1 相连，豚鼠接地。监听输出与扬声器连接。

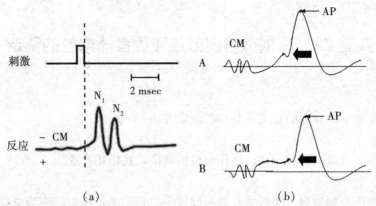

（a）短声刺激引起的微音器电位（CM）及耳蜗神经干动作电位（AP，包括 N_1、N_2 两个负电位）

（b）A 与 B 对比表明，声音位相改变时，CM 位相倒转，但 AP 位相没有变化

图 9-6　由短声刺激引起的微音器电位和听神经动作电位

【实验项目】

（1）对豚鼠外耳讲话、唱歌、鼓掌，听扬声器声音。

（2）观察声音刺激引起的耳蜗神经干动作电位。增加刺激器输出强度，当屏幕出现电位波动时，调节刺激器频率、扫描速度及灵敏度，使 CM 和 N_1、N_2 显示于屏幕上，辨别各波。

（3）改变声音刺激的强度，观察耳蜗微音器电位和听神经动作电位的变化。

（4）改变声音刺激的位相，观察耳蜗微音器电位和听神经动作电位的变化。

【注意事项】

（1）切勿使小骨钻插入鼓室过深而伤及耳蜗。

（2）实验中注意止血，避免血渗入耳蜗，影响信号的采集。

【思考与评价】

1. 耳蜗微音器电位有无潜伏期？

2. 比较耳蜗微音器电位与听神经动作电位的特点。

【英文专业单词】

微音器效应（microphonic effect）　微音器电位（cochlear microphonic potential，CM）

（彭碧文）

实验 30　人体眼震颤的观察

【实验目的】

（1）观察人体旋转停止后的眼震颤。

（2）了解内耳（internal ear）迷路机能。

【实验原理】

眼震颤（nystagmus）是躯体旋转运动时所引起的前庭反应中最特殊的一种表现形式。

当人体低头 30°围绕垂直轴进行旋转运动时，可使两侧水平半规管壶腹脊毛细胞(hair cell)受到不同的刺激，从而出现水平方向的震颤。当旋转停止后，由于内淋巴 (endolymph)流动方向的改变使两侧毛细胞受到的刺激改变，从而产生于旋转开始方向相反的眼震颤。

【实验对象】

人。

【实验药品与器材】

旋转椅。

【实验方法与步骤】

受试者坐在旋转椅上，闭目，头低 30°，以约 2s/周的速度做原地旋转 10~15 周，然后突然使旋转椅停止不动，受试者立即睁开双眼，实验者录制眼震颤的过程，并观察记录快动向、慢动向的方向和持续时间。

【注意事项】

受试者在进行旋转过程中，应注意保护，防止摔倒或碰伤。

【思考题】

1. 眼震颤的方向如何判断？

2. 眼震颤与旋转方向是什么关系？

【英文专业单词】

眼震颤(nystagmus)

（王　媛）

第 10 章 神 经 生 理

实验 31 反射时的测定与反射弧的分析

【实验思路与目的】

(1)通过蛙屈肌反射，分析反射弧的组成部分，反射弧的完整性与反射活动的关系。

(2)学习反射时的测定方法。

【实验原理】

反射是指在中枢神经系统的参与下，机体对外环境变化所做出的规律性的应答。反射活动的结构基础是反射弧，完整的反射弧包括感受器、传入神经、神经中枢、传出神经和效应器五部分，其中任一环节中断(结构和功能受到破坏)，反射弧活动就无法完成。反射时是指反射通过反射弧各部分所需的时间，刺激作用于感受器开始到效应器出现反射活动所经过的时间。

【实验对象】

蛙或蟾蜍。

【药品与器材】

任氏液、0.5%硫酸溶液、蛙类手术器械一套、玻璃平皿、小烧杯、铁支架、滴管、秒表、滤纸片($1cm^2$)、大头针、棉线、刺激电极。

【方法与步骤】

制备脊蟾蜍：取蛙或蟾蜍一只，用探针从枕骨大孔处刺入颅腔破坏脑组织；或者用粗剪刀由两侧口裂剪去头颅。用大头针做成的小钩钩住蛙的下颌，将其悬挂在铁支架上。

【实验项目】

1. 反射时的测定

用 0.5%硫酸刺激蛙足趾部的皮肤，用秒表测定从浸入硫酸到出现反射的时间。用清水洗干净足趾部皮肤，重复测定。测三次取平均值。

2. 反射弧的分析

(1)观察屈肌反射：用培养皿盛放 0.5%硫酸溶液 5ml，将蛙左后肢足趾尖浸入 0.5%硫酸溶液中，观察有无屈肌反射发生。

（2）去掉左后足趾部的皮肤再观察屈肌反射：在趾关节上方做一环形切口，将足趾部皮肤剥掉重复步骤（1），观察有无屈肌反射发生。

（3）按照步骤（1）将蛙右后足趾尖浸入 0.5% 硫酸溶液中，观察反射活动。

（4）剪断右侧坐骨神经：在右侧大腿背侧剪开皮肤，在股二头肌和半膜肌之间用玻璃分针分离坐骨神经，双结扎，在两结扎线间剪断神经。重复步骤（3）观察反射活动。

（5）电刺激右侧坐骨神经中枢端，观察腿部反应。

（6）电刺激右侧坐骨神经外周端，观察腿部反应。

（7）用探针捣毁脊髓后，重复步骤（3），观察反应。

【注意事项】

（1）捣毁脑部组织应当完全，避免部分脑组织保留，出现自主活动。

（2）每次实验浸入硫酸的部位深度应当相同，不宜太深。

（3）每次用硫酸刺激完毕后，应迅速用清水洗去残余硫酸，并擦干水渍，以免硫酸灼伤皮肤。

【思考与评价】

1. 本实验中屈肌反射反射弧包括哪些组成部分，实验中每一步分别影响哪一部分的结构和功能？

2. 反射时的长短主要由哪些因素决定？

【英文专业单词】

反射弧（reflex arc）　　　反射活动（reflex action）

反射时（reflex time）

（石俊枝）

实验 32　去大脑僵直

【实验目的】

观察去大脑僵直的现象，理解脑干对姿势的调节作用。

【实验原理】

适当的肌紧张对维持姿势十分重要。中枢神经系统对肌紧张有易化作用和抑制作用，从而使骨骼肌保持适当的紧张度，以维持姿势。当在动物中脑的上、下丘之间离断脑干，大脑皮层运动区和纹状体等部位与脑干网状结构的功能联系中断，肌紧张的抑制作用减弱，而易化作用相对增强，动物将出现肌肉强直的现象，表现为四肢僵直、头尾昂起，脊柱挺硬，这种现象称为去大脑僵直。

【实验对象】

家兔。

【实验药品与器材】

20% 乌拉坦、生理盐水、兔头固定架、咬骨钳、颅钻、脱脂棉球、刺激电极、纱布、哺乳动物手术器械。

1. 麻醉

从兔耳缘静脉按 0.5~0.8g/kg 缓慢注射 20%乌拉坦。

2. 手术操作

(1)将家兔俯卧位固定于兔头固定架，剪去头顶部的毛。

(2)从眉间至枕部沿头顶部正中切开皮肤，分离皮下组织及肌肉，并分离骨膜，暴露出颅骨。

(3)在矢状缝旁的颅顶部位用骨钻开孔。

(4)用咬骨钳扩大创口，暴露大脑皮层。当一侧大脑皮层已暴露后，将手术刀柄伸入矢状窦与颅骨之间，小心分离，然后用咬骨钳扩大骨创至暴露对侧大脑皮层。扩大创骨过程中勿损伤矢状窦，以免大出血。剪开硬脑膜，暴露大脑皮层表面。

(5)从大脑半球后缘轻轻翻开枕叶，即可见到四叠体(上、下丘)，用刀片在上、下丘之间向下颌角方向插入，将脑干完全离断。

【实验项目】

观察家兔四肢、颈部、背部及尾巴的姿势变化。若脑干切断部位准确，可见家兔出现四肢伸直、头昂起、尾上翘、脊柱挺硬等。若不明显，可用手提起兔的背部，抖动动物，动物四肢伸肌受重力牵拉，伸肌的肌紧张会明显增强。

【注意事项】

(1)动物麻醉宜浅，麻醉过深不易出现去大脑僵直的现象。

(2)手术过程中勿伤及矢状窦，避免大出血。

(3)横断脑干部位要准确，过低可能损伤延髓，导致呼吸停止；过高则不易出现去大脑僵直的现象。

【思考题】

产生去大脑僵直的机制是什么？

【英文专业单词】

去大脑僵直(decerebrate rigidity)

(王泽芬)

实验 33　皮层机能定位

【实验目的】

(1)观察电刺激家兔大脑皮层不同区域引起的肌肉运动。

(2)理解大脑皮层运动区的功能定位特点。

【实验原理】

大脑皮层是调节躯体运动的最高级中枢。大脑皮层运动区通过锥体系和锥体外系下行通路控制脊髓前角运动神经元、脑神经运动神经元的活动，以支配肌肉运动。对接受神经外科手术治疗的患者，通过电刺激大脑皮层不同区域，可以观察到皮层运动区不同部位引起的骨骼肌运动及其功能定位的特点。这种皮层运动区机能定位在较低等的动物如鼠、兔已具有一定的雏形，在高等灵长类动物及人类则更明显。

【实验对象】

家兔(体重 2~2.5kg)。

【实验药品与器材】

20%乌拉坦、生理盐水、液体石蜡、兔头固定架、咬骨钳、颅钻、脱脂棉球、刺激电极、骨蜡或止血海绵、BL-420E 生物信号采集系统、哺乳动物手术器械。

【实验方法】

1. 麻醉

从兔耳缘静脉按 0.8~1.0g/kg 缓慢注射 20%乌拉坦。

2. 手术操作

(1)将家兔俯卧位固定于兔头固定架，剪去头顶部的毛。

(2)从眉间至枕部沿头顶部正中切开皮肤，分离皮下组织及肌肉，并分离骨膜，暴露出颅骨。

(3)在矢状缝旁的颅顶部位用骨钻钻开颅骨(图 10-1)。

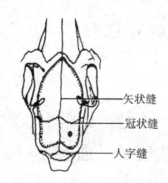

矢状缝
冠状缝
人字缝

图 10-1　兔颅骨标志示意(黑点为骨钻钻孔的位置)

(4)用咬骨钳扩大创口，暴露大脑皮层。当一侧大脑皮层已暴露后，将手术刀柄伸入矢状窦与颅骨之间，小心分离，然后用咬骨钳扩大骨创至暴露对侧大脑皮层。扩大创骨过程中勿损伤矢状窦，以免出血。

(5)剪开硬脑膜，暴露大脑皮层表面，并滴加 37℃液体石蜡以保护脑组织。

【实验项目】

接通刺激器的电源，选择合适的参数(波宽为 0.1~0.2ms，强度为 10~20V，频率为 20Hz)。将刺激电极与刺激器相连，依次刺激大脑皮层的不同区域，每次持续时间 5~10s，观察家兔的肌肉运动，将结果标记在事先画好的兔大脑半球示意图上，并与图 10-2 比较。

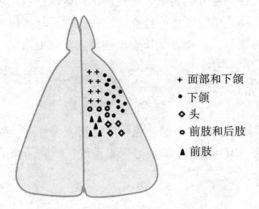

+ 面部和下颌

• 下颌

◇ 头

○ 前肢和后肢

▲ 前肢

图 10-2　兔大脑皮层运动区的刺激效应图

【注意事项】

(1)麻醉不宜过深，否则影响刺激的效应。

(2)扩大骨创过程中勿损伤矢状窦。若创口出血较多，可用骨蜡或止血棉球止血。

(3)注意保护大脑皮层。

【思考题】

大脑皮层运动功能定位有哪些特点？

【英文专业单词】

大脑皮层(cerebral cortex)

（王泽芬）

实验 34　血 脑 屏 障

【实验目的】

(1)学习检测血脑屏障通透性的方法。

(2)理解血脑屏障的生理作用。

【实验原理】

血脑屏障指存在于血液和脑组织之间的屏障，可限制物质在血液和脑组织中的自由交换。水和游离状态的脂溶性物质，如 CO_2、O_2 等很容易通过血脑屏障，非脂溶性的大分子物质不易通过。血脑屏障的结构基础是无孔或少孔的毛细血管内皮细胞，内皮下基底膜和星形胶质细胞的血管周足等结构。血脑屏障的存在对保持脑组织化学环境的稳定和防止血液中有害物质侵入脑内具有重要的生理意义。

台盼蓝是一种细胞活性染料，其分子量(MW 916 Da)及亲水性使其不易通过血脑屏障。因此，台盼蓝是一种检测血脑屏障通透性的常用染料。

【实验对象】

小白鼠。

【实验药品与器材】

乙醚、1ml 无菌注射器、1%台盼蓝溶液、眼科剪子和镊子。

【实验方法】

(1)将小鼠放入内有浸有乙醚棉球的烧杯中进行吸入麻醉。

(2)用 1ml 无菌注射器腹腔注射 1%台盼蓝溶液 1ml，或尾静脉注射 1%台盼蓝溶液 0.5ml。

(3)观察小鼠皮肤，尤其是眼、嘴的颜色变化。当眼、嘴颜色变蓝时，由头到尾沿背中线剪开皮肤，暴露皮下、肌肉和内脏，观察颜色变化；小心剖开颅骨和椎骨，暴露脑和脊髓，与皮下、肌肉及内脏比较。比较台盼蓝注射小鼠与正常小鼠有何不同。

【思考题】

1. 为什么台盼蓝注射小鼠的内脏变蓝，但大脑、脊髓不变蓝色？

2. 试述血脑屏障有何生理作用？

【英文专业单词】

血脑屏障(blood-brain barrier)

（王泽芬）

实验 35　损伤小鼠一侧小脑对躯体运动的影响

【实验目的】

观察小鼠一侧小脑损伤后对躯体活动的影响。

【实验原理】

小脑是参与运动调控的重要中枢之一。小脑本身并不发动运动，但在运动的策划及运动程序的编制、运动的协调中发挥重要作用。小脑可分为三个主要功能部分：①前庭小脑参与身体姿势平衡功能的调节；②脊髓小脑能有效利用来自大脑运动皮层和外周感觉的反馈信息来调节进行过程中的运动，协助大脑皮层对随意运动进行适时的调控；③皮层小脑与运动的策划、运动程序的编制有关。小脑损伤后并不引起任何肌肉麻痹，但可出现随意运动失调、平衡失调及站立不稳等表现。

【实验对象】

小白鼠。

【实验药品与器材】

乙醚、手术剪、脱脂棉球、镊子、大头针、烧杯。

【实验方法】

1. 麻醉

将小鼠放入内有浸有乙醚棉球的烧杯中进行吸入麻醉。

2. 手术操作

（1）从正中线剪开头部皮肤至枕部，钝性剥离皮下组织和肌肉，暴露颅骨。

（2）仔细辨认小鼠颅骨的骨缝，右手持大头针在人字缝后 1mm，正中线旁开 2mm 刺入（图 10-3），深度 3mm，然后以前后方向搬动针尖数次，一徘徊一侧小脑部分。取出大头针，棉球按压止血。

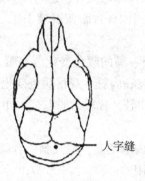

人字缝

图 10-3　破坏小鼠小脑的位置示意图（黑点为大头针刺入处）

【实验项目】

待小鼠清醒后，观察小白鼠身体是否向一侧旋转或翻滚，两侧肢体的肌张力是否一样。

【注意事项】

（1）针刺入不能过深，以免损伤延髓。

（2）如小鼠症状不明显，可能由于小脑破坏不完全，可在原刺入处重新损毁一次。

【思考题】

一侧小脑损伤后动物的姿势和躯体运动有何变化？

【英文专业单词】

小脑损伤（cerebellum injury）

（王泽芬）

实验 36　肱二头肌反射

【实验目的】

学习肱二头肌反射的方法。

【实验原理】

检查腱反射是临床了解神经系统功能状态的最客观的评价方式。肱二头肌反射是指叩击肱二头肌腱，产生屈肘的反射。传入神经为肌皮神经内的感觉纤维，反射中枢为颈 5~6 脊髓灰质，传出神经为肌皮神经的躯体运动纤维，效应器为肱二头肌。

【实验对象】

　　人。

【实验器材】

　　叩诊锤。

【实验步骤】

　　(1)确定肱二头肌肌腱所在部位：让受试者屈曲右侧肘部，以拇指触诊肘窝，可触及肘窝部位突出的粗条索状肱二头肌肌腱。

　　(2)检查者用左手拖住受试者右侧肘部，将上臂和前臂成稍大于90°屈曲，肱二头肌需保持放松状态。

　　(3)为确保叩诊锤准确叩击在肌腱上，而不是叩击在肌肉上，检查者以左拇指按在受试者右侧肘部肱二头肌肌腱上，用叩诊锤叩击检查者左拇指。正常反应为肱二头肌收缩，表现为前臂快速的屈曲动作。

【注意事项】

　　受试者需保持精神放松、四肢肌肉松弛。

【英文专业单词】

　　肱二头肌反射(biceps reflex)

（张先荣）

实验 37　膝 跳 反 射

【实验原理】

　　膝跳反射是快速叩击髌骨下方的髌韧带，使小腿做急速前踢的动作。当快速叩击髌骨下方的髌韧带时，股四头肌(伸肌)受到快速牵拉，其内的肌梭兴奋，神经冲动传向脊髓并兴奋脊髓内 α 运动神经元，引起被牵拉肌肉(即股四头肌)的收缩；同时肌梭传入冲动通过传入侧支性抑制引起股后肌群(屈肌)的舒张，引起小腿前踢。

　　膝跳反射属于腱反射，是单突触反射。腱反射不能引出或反射亢进，均为异常。

【实验对象】

　　人。

【实验器材】

　　叩诊锤。

【实验方法】

　　(1)被检测者采取坐位，被检测下肢自然地搭在另一下肢上，使膝关节半屈，小腿自由下垂。

　　(2)实验者用叩诊锤快速地叩击被检测下肢膝盖下方的髌韧带，观察小腿的反应(图10-4)。

（王泽芬）

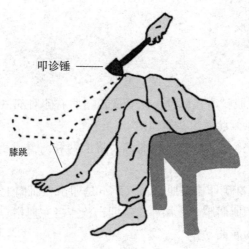

图 10-4　漆跳反射

实验 38　跟 腱 反 射

【实验目的】

　　熟悉几种人体腱反射的检查方法。

【实验原理】

　　牵张反射是最简单的躯体运动反射，包括肌紧张和腱反射两种类型。腱反射是指快速牵拉肌腱时发生的牵张反射。腱反射是一种单突触反射，其感受器是肌梭，中枢在脊髓前角，效应器主要是肌肉收缩较快的快肌纤维成分。腱反射的减弱或消退，常提示反射弧的传入、传出通路或脊髓反射中枢的损害或中断；而腱反射的亢进，则提示高位中枢的病变。因此，临床上常通过检查腱反射来了解神经系统的功能状态。

【实验对象】

　　人。

【药品与器材】

　　叩诊槌。

【方法与步骤】

　　受试者应予以充分合作，避免精神紧张和意识性控制，四肢保持对称、放松。如果受试者精神或注意力集中于检查部位，可使反射受到抑制。此时，可用加强法予以消除。最简单的加强法是叫受试者主动收缩所要检查反射以外的其他肌肉。

【实验项目】

　　(1)肱二头肌反射：受试者取端坐位，检查者用左手托住受试者右肘部，左前臂托住受试者的前臂，并以左手拇指按于受试者的右肘部肱二头肌肌腱上，然后用叩诊槌叩击检查者自己的左拇指。正常反应为肱二头肌收缩，表现为前臂呈快速的屈曲动作。

（2）肱三头肌反射：受试者上臂稍外展，前臂及上臂半屈成90°。检查者以左手托住其右肘部内侧，然后用叩诊槌轻叩尺骨鹰嘴的上方1~2cm处的肱三头肌肌腱。正常反应为肱三头肌收缩，表现为前臂呈伸展运动。

（3）膝反射：受试者取坐位，双小腿自然下垂悬空。检查者以右手持叩诊槌，轻叩膝盖下股四头肌肌腱。正常反应为小腿伸直动作。

（4）跟腱反射：受试者跪于椅子上，下肢于膝关节部位呈直角屈曲，踝关节以下悬空。检查者以叩诊槌轻叩跟腱。正常反应为腓肠肌收缩，足向跖面屈曲。

【注意事项】

（1）检查者动作轻缓，消除受检者紧张情绪，四肢肌肉放松。

（2）每次叩击的部位要准确，叩击的力度要适中。

【思考与评价】

以膝反射为例，说明从叩击股四头肌肌腱到引起小腿伸直动作的全过程。

【英文专业单词】

跟腱反射(achilles tendon reflex)

（陈桃香）

参考文献

[1]朱大年，王庭槐主编. 生理学[M]. 8 版. 北京：人民卫生出版社，2013.

[2]姚泰主编. 生理学(供 8 年制及 7 年制临床医学等专业用)[M]. 北京：人民卫生出版社，2010.

[3]孙久荣，黄玉芝主编. 生理学实验[M]. 北京：北京大学出版社，2005.

[4]王庭槐主编. 生理学实验教程[M]. 北京：北京大学医学出版社，2004.

[5]胡还忠主编. 医学机能学实验教程[M]. 北京：科学出版社，2014.